TRB SPECIAL
REPORT
282

Does the Built Environment Influence

Physical Activity?

EXAMINING THE EVIDENCE

Committee on Physical Activity, Health,
Transportation, and Land Use

TRANSPORTATION RESEARCH BOARD
INSTITUTE OF MEDICINE
OF THE NATIONAL ACADEMIES

Transportation Research Board
Washington, D.C.
2005
www.TRB.org

Transportation Research Board Special Report 282

Subscriber Category
IA planning and administration

Transportation Research Board publications are available by ordering individual publications directly from the TRB Business Office, through the Internet at www.TRB.org or national-academies.org/trb, or by annual subscription through organizational or individual affiliation with TRB. Affiliates and library subscribers are eligible for substantial discounts. For further information, contact the Transportation Research Board Business Office, 500 Fifth Street, NW, Washington, DC 20001 (telephone 202-334-3213; fax 202-334-2519; or e-mail TRBsales@nas.edu).

NOTICE: The project that is the subject of this report was approved by the Governing Board of the National Research Council, whose members are drawn from the councils of the National Academy of Sciences, the National Academy of Engineering, and the Institute of Medicine. The members of the committee responsible for the report were chosen for their special competencies and with regard for appropriate balance.

This report has been reviewed by a group other than the authors according to the procedures approved by a Report Review Committee consisting of members of the National Academy of Sciences, the National Academy of Engineering, and the Institute of Medicine.

This study was sponsored by the Robert Wood Johnson Foundation and the Centers for Disease Control and Prevention.

Cover design by Tony Olivis, Circle Graphics.

Library of Congress Cataloging-in-Publication Data

Does the built environment influence physical activity? : examining the evidence /
    Committee on Physical Activity, Health, Transportation, and Land Use, Transportation
    Research Board, Institute of Medicine of the National Academies.
        p. cm.—(Special report ; 282)
    ISBN 0-309-09498-4
    1. Urban health. 2. Transportation—Health aspects. 3. Health behavior. 4. Physical
    fitness. 5. Exercise. I. National Research Council (U.S.). Committee on Physical
    Activity, Health, Transportation, and Land Use. II. National Research Council (U.S.).
    Transportation Research Board. III. Institute of Medicine (U.S.). IV. Special report
    (National Research Council (U.S.). Transportation Research Board) ; 282.

    RA566.7.D646 2005
    362.1'042—dc22

                                                                2005041846

THE NATIONAL ACADEMIES
Advisers to the Nation on Science, Engineering, and Medicine

The **National Academy of Sciences** is a private, nonprofit, self-perpetuating society of distinguished scholars engaged in scientific and engineering research, dedicated to the furtherance of science and technology and to their use for the general welfare. On the authority of the charter granted to it by the Congress in 1863, the Academy has a mandate that requires it to advise the federal government on scientific and technical matters. Dr. Bruce M. Alberts is president of the National Academy of Sciences.

The **National Academy of Engineering** was established in 1964, under the charter of the National Academy of Sciences, as a parallel organization of outstanding engineers. It is autonomous in its administration and in the selection of its members, sharing with the National Academy of Sciences the responsibility for advising the federal government. The National Academy of Engineering also sponsors engineering programs aimed at meeting national needs, encourages education and research, and recognizes the superior achievements of engineers. Dr. William A. Wulf is president of the National Academy of Engineering.

The **Institute of Medicine** was established in 1970 by the National Academy of Sciences to secure the services of eminent members of appropriate professions in the examination of policy matters pertaining to the health of the public. The Institute acts under the responsibility given to the National Academy of Sciences by its congressional charter to be an adviser to the federal government and, on its own initiative, to identify issues of medical care, research, and education. Dr. Harvey V. Fineberg is president of the Institute of Medicine.

The **National Research Council** was organized by the National Academy of Sciences in 1916 to associate the broad community of science and technology with the Academy's purposes of furthering knowledge and advising the federal government. Functioning in accordance with general policies determined by the Academy, the Council has become the principal operating agency of both the National Academy of Sciences and the National Academy of Engineering in providing services to the government, the public, and the scientific and engineering communities. The Council is administered jointly by both the Academies and the Institute of Medicine. Dr. Bruce M. Alberts and Dr. William A. Wulf are chair and vice chair, respectively, of the National Research Council.

The **Transportation Research Board** is a division of the National Research Council, which serves the National Academy of Sciences and the National Academy of Engineering. The Board's mission is to promote innovation and progress in transportation through research. In an objective and interdisciplinary setting, the Board facilitates the sharing of information on transportation practice and policy by researchers and practitioners; stimulates research and offers research management services that promote technical excellence; provides expert advice on transportation policy and programs; and disseminates research results broadly and encourages their implementation. The Board's varied activities annually engage more than 5,000 engineers, scientists, and other transportation researchers and practitioners from the public and private sectors and academia, all of whom contribute their expertise in the public interest. The program is supported by state transportation departments, federal agencies including the component administrations of the U.S. Department of Transportation, and other organizations and individuals interested in the development of transportation. **www.TRB.org**

www.national-academies.org

Committee on Physical Activity, Health, Transportation, and Land Use

Susan Hanson, Clark University, Worcester, Massachusetts, *Chair*
Bobbie A. Berkowitz, University of Washington, Seattle, *Vice Chair*
Barbara E. Ainsworth, San Diego State University, San Diego, California
Steven N. Blair, Cooper Institute, Dallas, Texas
Robert B. Cervero, University of California, Berkeley
Donald D. T. Chen, Smart Growth America, Washington, D.C.
Randall Crane, University of California, Los Angeles
Mindy Thompson Fullilove, Columbia University, New York
Genevieve Giuliano, University of Southern California, Los Angeles
T. Keith Lawton, Metro, Portland, Oregon (retired)
Patricia L. Mokhtarian, University of California, Davis
Kenneth E. Powell, Georgia Department of Human Resources, Atlanta
Jane C. Stutts, University of North Carolina, Chapel Hill
Richard P. Voith, Econsult Corporation, Philadelphia, Pennsylvania

National Research Council Staff
Nancy P. Humphrey, *Study Director,* Transportation Research Board
Carrie I. Szlyk, *Program Officer,* Institute of Medicine

Preface

Public health officials have long been concerned about the effect of the environment on human health. In the nineteenth century, public health efforts in the United States were focused on controlling the spread of infectious disease, and advances in sanitation and the provision of clean water contributed to improvements in the health of the population. At the turn of the century, urban reformers adopted zoning laws and building codes to reduce the spread of disease from overcrowded conditions in central cities by lowering housing densities, as well as to separate residences from noxious commercial and industrial enterprises. Today, public health efforts are focused on the prevention of chronic disease, and the question has arisen of whether the decentralized and largely automobile-dependent development patterns that emerged in part in response to earlier public health concerns are contributing to the increasingly sedentary lifestyles of the U.S. population—a known risk factor for many chronic illnesses.

In this context, the Robert Wood Johnson Foundation and the Centers for Disease Control and Prevention requested the present study to examine the connection between the built environment and the physical activity levels of the U.S. population. In response to this request, the Transportation Research Board (TRB) and the Institute of Medicine (IOM) formed a committee consisting of 14 experts from the transportation and public health communities. The panel was chaired by Susan Hanson, Landry University Professor and Director of the Graduate School of Geography at Clark University and a member of the National Academy of Sciences. Bobbie Berkowitz, Professor and Chair of the Department of

Psychosocial and Community Health at the University of Washington's School of Nursing and an IOM member, served as vice chair. The expertise of the panel members lies in such diverse fields as transportation demand and travel behavior, land use planning and regulation, public health, physical activity and education, economics and public policy, safety, and social and behavioral science research and methods.

To carry out its charge, the committee commissioned several papers to explore various aspects of the relationships among land use, transportation, and physical activity. The first set of three papers was written by Ross C. Brownson and Tegan Boehmer, School of Public Health, St. Louis University; Susan L. Handy, Department of Environmental Science and Policy, University of California at Davis; and Marlon G. Boarnet, Department of Planning, Policy, and Design, University of California at Irvine. These papers, respectively, examine long-term trends in land use patterns, travel behavior, employment and occupation, and time use that are related to physical activity levels; critically review the literature on these relationships, in particular for evidence of causal connections; and elaborate on the methodological and data challenges facing researchers in this area. The second set of three papers was authored by Susan D. Kirby, Kirby Marketing Solutions, Inc., and Marla Hollander, Leadership for Active Living program, San Diego State University; Anastasia Loukaitou-Sideris, School of Public Policy and Research, University of California at Los Angeles; and Michael D. Meyer and Eric Dumbaugh, School of Civil and Environmental Engineering, Georgia Institute of Technology. These papers examine the role of intervening variables that may influence individual preferences for physical activity, as well as available opportunities and choices. They address, respectively, the role of social marketing in shaping individual preferences and behavior; the importance of safety and security, both perceived and actual; and institutional and regulatory forces that affect what is built and where. The final paper, by Elliott D. Sclar, Urban Planning Program, Columbia University, and Mary E. Northridge and Emily Karpel, Mailman School of Public Health, also Columbia University, examines educational programs that link the fields of public health and urban planning for the purpose of training future researchers and professionals, with a focus on the need for interdisciplinary curricula and training.

All seven papers underwent extensive review and comment by the committee and were revised numerous times. They are listed in Appendix A, along with the addresses where they can be accessed on the Internet. The reader is cautioned that the interpretations and conclusions drawn in the papers are those of their authors; the key findings endorsed by the committee appear in the body of this report.

The committee also drew from a paper on the role of segregation and poverty in limiting choices for physical activity among disadvantaged populations, written by Benjamin P. Bowser, Department of Sociology and Social Services, California State University at Hayward. Dr. Bowser raised many important issues that stimulated discussion among the committee and at a workshop (see below) regarding the special problems of physical activity for these populations. Many of these issues are covered in this report.

Recognizing that the above papers could not fully represent the relatively new but rapidly growing field of research linking the built environment to physical activity levels, the committee held a workshop midway through the project to involve a broader audience of experts drawn from academia, consulting firms, professional associations, advocacy groups, state and federal agencies, congressional staff, and the press. At this workshop, each paper was presented and critiqued by a commentator, then discussed by the invited participants. The workshop concluded with a wrap-up by two rapporteurs—one from the physical activity and one from the transportation community. Of the more than 160 individuals invited to the workshop, 46 attended in addition to the committee, commentators, rapporteurs, and staff. Their names and affiliations, along with the workshop agenda, can be found in Appendix B. The commentary and critiques offered during the workshop were considered in both finalizing the authored papers and preparing this final report.

The committee also supplemented its expertise by receiving briefings at its meetings from a wide range of experts. In particular, the committee thanks Robert T. Best, President of Westar Associates, and Thomas Lee, former CEO of the Newhall Land and Farming Company—two California developers who discussed their experience with building large planned communities amenable to walking and cycling. The committee also thanks Donald H. Pickrell, Chief Economist at the U.S. Department of Transportation's John A. Volpe National Transportation Systems Center, for his presentation on requirements for establishing the connections among urban form, travel, and physical activity; Karla Henderson, Professor and Chair, Department of Recreation and Leisure Studies, University of North Carolina at Chapel Hill, who spoke on the role of recreational facilities in increasing physical activity; Roland Sturm, Senior Economist, the RAND Corporation, for his presentation on the economics of physical inactivity; and Leslie S. Linton, Deputy Director of Active Living Research, a program funded by the Robert Wood Johnson Foundation and housed at San Diego State University, for her update on program-sponsored research related to this study.

This report has been reviewed in draft form by individuals chosen for their diverse perspectives and technical expertise, in accordance with procedures approved by the National Research Council's (NRC's) Report Review Committee. The purpose of this independent review is to provide candid and critical comments that assist the authors and NRC in making the published report as sound as possible and to ensure that the report meets institutional standards for objectivity, evidence, and responsiveness to the study charge. The content of the review comments and draft manuscript remain confidential to protect the integrity of the deliberative process. The committee thanks the following individuals for their participation in the review of this report: Hank Dittmar, Reconnecting America, Las Vegas, New Mexico; Robert Dunphy, Urban Land Institute, Washington, D.C.; Jonathan Fielding, Department of Health Services, Los Angeles County, California; William Fischel, Dartmouth College, Hanover, New Hampshire; Lester Hoel, University of Virginia, Charlottesville; Russell Pate, University of South Carolina, Columbia; Joseph Schofer, Northwestern University, Evanston, Illinois; Boyd Swinburn, Deakin University, Melbourne, Australia; and Martin Wachs, University of California, Berkeley.

Although the reviewers listed above provided many constructive comments and suggestions, they were not asked to endorse the committee's conclusions or recommendations, nor did they see the final draft of the report before its release. The review of this report was overseen by Enriqueta C. Bond, Burroughs Wellcome Fund, and C. Michael Walton, University of Texas at Austin. Appointed by NRC, they were responsible for making certain that an independent examination of the report was carried out in accordance with institutional procedures and that all review comments were carefully considered. Responsibility for the final content of this report rests entirely with the authoring committee and the institution.

Nancy P. Humphrey of TRB, together with Carrie I. Szlyk of IOM, managed the study. Both drafted sections of the final report under the guidance of the committee and the supervision of Stephen R. Godwin, Director of Studies and Information Services at TRB, and Rose Martinez, Director of the Board on Health Promotion and Disease Prevention at IOM. Suzanne Schneider, Associate Executive Director of TRB, managed the report review process. Special appreciation is expressed to Rona Briere, who edited the report. Amelia Mathis assisted with meeting arrangements and communications with committee members, Jocelyn Sands handled contracting with the paper authors, and Alisa Decatur provided word processing support for preparation of the final manuscript. In the TRB Publications Office, Jennifer Weeks prepared the final manuscript and the commissioned papers for posting on the web; Norman Solomon provided final editorial guidance; and Juanita Green managed the book design and production, under the supervision of Javy Awan.

Glossary

Accelerometer. A monitoring device that measures the intensity of an activity.

Accessibility. Distance to or from destinations or facilities.

Body mass index (BMI). One of the most commonly used measures for defining overweight and obesity, calculated as weight in pounds divided by the square of height in inches, multiplied by 703.

Built environment. Defined broadly to include land use patterns, the transportation system, and design features that together provide opportunities for travel and physical activity. *Land use patterns* refer to the spatial distribution of human activities. The *transportation system* refers to the physical infrastructure and services that provide the spatial links or connectivity among activities. *Design* refers to the aesthetic, physical, and functional qualities of the built environment, such as the design of buildings and streetscapes, and relates to both land use patterns and the transportation system.

Case-control studies. Studies in which exposure to an acknowledged risk factor is compared between individuals from the same population with and without a condition. For example, individuals could be sorted on the basis of their activity level (e.g., active versus sedentary) into case and control groups to see whether there are statistically significant differences in environmental characteristics that may influence the propensity of the two groups to be physically active.

Connectivity. The directness of travel to destinations.

Context-sensitive design. A project development process encompassing geometric design that attempts to address safety and efficiency while being responsive to or consistent with a road's natural and human environment.

Cross-sectional studies. Studies that examine the relationship between conditions (e.g., physical activity behaviors) and other variables of interest in a defined population at a single point in time. Cross-sectional studies can quantify the presence and magnitude of associations between variables. Unlike longitudinal studies, however, they cannot be used to determine the temporal relationship between variables, and evidence of cause and effect cannot be assumed.

Cul-de-sac. A street, lane, or passage closed at one end.

Decentralization. Movement of population and employment away from city centers.

Deconcentration. Movement of population and employment to less-dense areas.

Demand theory. Derived from economics and psychology, posits that individuals make decisions in their self-interest, given the option to do so. In other words, most choices are made on the basis of their feasibility and their relative costs and benefits to the individual. Thus, for example, one would assume that people would be more likely to walk if walking trips became more pleasant, safer, or in any sense easier, or if alternatives to walking became more costly or more difficult.

Density. Typically measured as employment or population per square mile.

Ecological models. Based on social cognitive theory, which explains behavior in terms of reciprocal relationships among the characteristics of a person, the person's behavior, and the environment in which the behavior is performed. Ecological models emphasize the role of the physical as well as the social environment.

Edge cities. A term coined by *Washington Post* journalist and author Joel Garreau in 1991 that refers to suburban cities, typically located near major freeway intersections.

Energy expenditure. Represents the sum of three factors: (*a*) resting energy expenditure to maintain basic body functions (approximately 60 percent of total energy requirements); (*b*) processing of food, which includes the thermic effect of digestion, absorption, transport, and deposition of nutrients (about 10 percent of total requirements); and (*c*) nonresting energy expenditure, primarily in the form of physical activity (about 30 percent of total requirements).

Energy imbalance. The situation that occurs when energy intake (calories consumed) exceeds or is less than total daily energy expenditure. Weight gain occurs when energy intake exceeds total daily energy expenditure for a prolonged period.

Exercise. A subcategory of physical activity defined as that which is planned, structured, repetitive, and purposive in the sense that improvement or maintenance of one or more components of physical fitness is the objective.

Experimental studies. Studies in which subjects are randomly assigned to the exposures of interest and followed for the outcome of interest. The most persuasive scientific evidence of causality usually is derived from experimental studies of individuals. The important advantages of experimental studies are that researchers have considerable control over all aspects of the study, including the type of exposure, the selection of subjects, and the assignment of exposure to the subjects.

Geographic information system (GIS). An automated system for the capture, storage, retrieval, analysis, and display of spatial data.

Global Positioning System (GPS). A worldwide radionavigation system comprising a constellation of 24 satellites and their ground stations. GPS uses these "man-made stars" as reference points to calculate positions accurate to a matter of meters.

Health. A state of complete physical, mental, and social well-being, not merely the absence of disease or infirmity.

Land use mix. Diversity or variety of land uses (e.g., residential, commercial, industrial).

Longitudinal studies. Studies in which individuals are known to have various levels of exposure and are followed over time to determine the incidence of outcomes. Quasi-experimental designs and natural experiments are two categories of longitudinal studies. Quasi-experimental designs are those in which the exposure is assigned but not according to a randomized experimental protocol. Investigators lack full control over the dose, timing, or allocation of subjects, but conduct the study as if it were an experiment. Natural experiments are situations in which different groups in a population have differing exposures and can be observed for different outcomes. Neither type of design is really an experiment because researchers have not randomly assigned the individuals to exposure groups.

Metabolic equivalent (MET). A unit used to estimate the metabolic cost (oxygen consumption) of physical activity. Activities that raise the rate of energy expenditure are frequently expressed as the ratio of working to resting metabolic rate.

Metropolitan statistical area (MSA). A statistical geographic entity consisting of at least one core urbanized area with a population of 50,000 or more. The MSA comprises the central county or counties containing the core and adjacent outlying counties with a high degree of social and economic integration with the central county, as measured through commuting ties with the counties containing the core.

Neotraditional developments. Developments whose design is characterized by land use and street patterns that encourage walking and cycling. These include such features as interconnected street networks, sidewalks, walking and cycling paths, mixed land uses, and higher densities than those of more typical suburban developments. Also known as *new-urbanist* developments.

Nonmotorized travel. Travel by nonmotorized means, including walking, cycling, small-wheeled transport (e.g., skates, skateboards, push scooters, hand carts), and wheelchair.

Obesity and overweight. Adults are defined as being obese if they have a body mass index (BMI) of 30 or greater, and as being overweight if they have a BMI of 25 but less than 30. Children and adolescents are defined as overweight if they have a BMI above the 95th percentile for their age and sex. A definition of obesity for children and adolescents on the basis of health outcomes or risk factors has not yet been formulated.

Overlay district. A planning tool that provides for special zoning requirements that are tailored to the characteristics of a particular area (e.g., special architectural character) or complementary to a particular public policy (e.g., higher-density building near rail transit stations) and are an exception to the underlying zoning.

Pedometer. A monitoring device that counts steps and measures distance.

Physical activity. Bodily movement produced by the contraction of skeletal muscle that increases energy expenditure above the basal (i.e., resting) level.

Physical fitness. The ability to carry out daily tasks with vigor and alertness, without undue fatigue, and with ample energy to enjoy leisure-time pursuits and to respond to unforeseen emergencies. Attributes of physical fitness include such characteristics as cardiorespiratory endurance; flexibility; balance; body composition; and muscular endurance, strength, and power.

Self-selection bias. In lay terms, refers to the need to distinguish the roles of personal attitudes, preferences, and motivations from external influences on observed behavior. For example, do people walk more in a particular neighborhood because of pleasant tree-lined sidewalks, or do they live in a neighborhood with pleasant tree-lined sidewalks because they like to walk? If researchers do not properly address this issue by identifying and separating these effects, their empirical results will be biased in the sense that features of the built environment may appear to influence physical activity more than they in fact do. (See Chapter 5 for a more technical definition of self-selection bias.)

Social marketing. The application of commercial marketing techniques to the analysis, planning, execution, and evaluation of programs designed to influence the voluntary behavior of target audiences, with the aim of improving their personal welfare and that of their society.

Traffic calming. Measures that attempt to slow traffic speeds in residential neighborhoods and near schools and pedestrian ways through physical devices designed to be self-enforcing. These include vertical deflections (speed humps and bumps and raised intersections); horizontal deflections (serpentines, bends, and deviations in a road); road narrowing (via neckdowns and chokers); and medians, central islands, and traffic circles.

Transit-oriented developments. Projects that involve mixed-use development (i.e., residential and commercial) near public transit stations.

Contents

Executive Summary

Physical activity is the leading health indicator in *Healthy People 2010*, a national agenda for reducing the most significant preventable threats to health. The scientific evidence is strong that regular physical activity—even at moderate levels, such as walking briskly for 30 minutes on 5 or more days per week—reduces the risk of premature mortality and the development of numerous chronic diseases, improves psychological well-being, and helps prevent weight gain and obesity by keeping caloric intake in balance with energy expenditure. Yet despite the scientific evidence, Americans have not taken sufficient initiative to meet federal guidelines on appropriate levels of total daily physical activity. Fully 55 percent of the U.S. adult population fall short of the guidelines, and approximately 25 percent report being completely inactive when not at work. Nearly one-third of high-school-age teenagers report not meeting recommended levels of physical activity, and 10 percent classify themselves as inactive. No corresponding summary assessment exists for children.

STUDY CONTEXT AND CHARGE

Over the past half-century or longer, major technological innovations—automation and the consequent decline of physically active occupations, labor-saving devices in the home, and the dominance of the automobile for personal travel—have substantially reduced the physical requirements of daily life. In addition, the steady decentralization of metropolitan area population and employment to low-density, widely dispersed suburban locations has increased travel distances to many destinations (e.g., schools, neighborhood shopping, transit stops) and made the private vehicle the most practical and convenient transport mode. Lifestyle and cultural changes, such as increases in television watching and other sedentary activities, have also played a role in reducing physical activity.

The built environment has recently come under scrutiny as an important potential contributor to reduced levels of physical activity. The purpose of this study is to contribute to the debate on this issue by examining the role of land use and travel patterns in the physical activity levels of the U.S. population. The charge to the study committee was to review the broad trends affecting the relationships among physical activity, health, transportation, and land use; summarize what is known about these relationships, including the strength and magnitude of any causal connections; draw implications for policy; and recommend priorities for future research. The built environment is broadly defined to include land use patterns, the transportation system, and design features that together provide opportunities for travel and physical activity.[1] Physical activity is defined as bodily movement produced by the contraction of skeletal muscle that increases energy expenditure above the basal level.

The built environment can be studied at various geographic scales—from the building and site to the neighborhood and regional levels. The focus of this study is primarily at the latter two levels; very little is known about physical activity at the building or site level. For the purposes of this study, physical activity is categorized into four types: leisure time or recreational, transportation, household, and occupational. The committee's interest is in the effect of the built environment on overall physical activity because total daily physical activity levels are what matter from a public

---

[1] *Land use patterns* refers to the spatial distribution of human activities. The *transportation system* refers to the physical infrastructure and services that provide the spatial links or connectivity among activities. *Design* refers to the aesthetic, physical, and functional qualities of the built environment, such as the design of buildings and streetscapes, and relates to both land use patterns and the transportation system.

health perspective, not whether an individual drives rather than walks or cycles on particular trips.

BENEFITS OF PHYSICAL ACTIVITY

The primary motivation for recent concern about inadequate levels of physical activity derives from the well-established, scientifically based causal connection between physical activity and health, as articulated in the U.S. Surgeon General's first report on *Physical Activity and Health* in 1996. That report and the results of subsequent research confirm that regular physical activity reduces the risk of premature mortality from all causes. Moreover, regular physical activity reduces the risk of developing several leading chronic illnesses, including cardiovascular disease (e.g., heart attacks, strokes), colon cancer, and non-insulin-dependent diabetes, as well as their precursors (e.g., high blood pressure, hypertension). Other benefits of physical activity include reductions in the risk of developing obesity, osteoporosis, and depression, and improvements in psychological well-being and quality of life.

Concern about low levels of physical activity stems from economic considerations as well. According to the Centers for Disease Control and Prevention, the direct medical expenses associated with physical inactivity totaled more than $76 billion in 2000. This figure does not take into account indirect costs, such as lost productivity from the physical and mental disabilities to which sedentary behavior contributes.

The problem of inadequate physical activity is frequently and mistakenly confused with obesity, particularly in the popular press. The recent marked rise in obesity levels among the U.S. population—a major public health concern—is due to an energy imbalance. Weight gain occurs when energy intake (calories consumed) exceeds total daily energy expenditure for a prolonged period. An important function of physical activity is energy expenditure, which helps maintain energy balance and keep weight gain in check. Addressing the obesity problem requires examining both energy intake (nutrition) and energy expenditure (physical activity). This study is focused on inadequate levels of physical activity—a major public health problem in its own right—and on the extent to which the built environment may play a role in fostering sedentary behavior.

ROLE OF THE BUILT ENVIRONMENT

The built environment is one of many variables thought to affect physical activity levels. The conceptual framework for this study (Figure ES-1) recognizes the complex relationships that affect the decision to be physically active. Much remains to be learned, however, about the relative importance of the individual (e.g., physical capacity, attitudes, preferences, time demands), the social context (e.g., social norms, support networks), and the physical environment as determinants of physically active behavior.

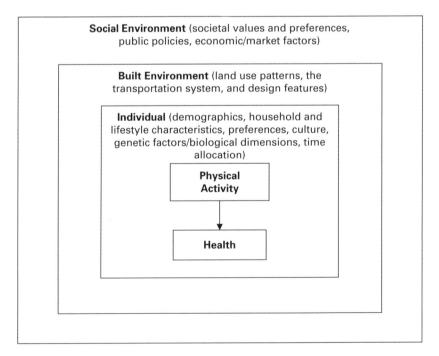

FIGURE ES-1 Overview of conceptual model for the study.

In contrast to the well-documented causal connection between physical activity and health, the role of the built environment in physical activity levels is a relatively new area of inquiry. The literature in this area is at an early stage of development, although it is growing rapidly. Results of this research to date, which has been largely cross-sectional, provide a growing body of evidence that shows an association between the built environment and physical activity levels. The science, however, is not sufficiently advanced to support causal connections or to identify with certainty those characteristics of the built environment most closely associated with physical activity behavior. Thus, the committee is unable to provide specific policy guidance, although it offers several recommendations for strengthening theory, research, and data that should provide a firmer basis for future policy making and intervention. The committee presents its consensus findings, conclusions, and recommendations in the following sections, which reflect the papers commissioned for this study, input provided at a workshop, numerous briefings provided to the committee at its meetings, and the expertise and judgment of its members.

FINDINGS

Physical activity levels have declined sharply over the past half-century because of reduced physical demands of work, household management, and travel, together with increased sedentary uses of free time. Labor-saving technological innovations have brought comfort, convenience, and time for more leisure activities. They have also resulted in more sedentary lifestyles with adverse health effects for many Americans. Changes in land use and travel may also have contributed to the decline in physical activity levels, but the specific contribution that the built environment could make in rebuilding physical activity into the daily routine is not well understood.

The built environment can facilitate or constrain physical activity. The built environment can be structured in ways that give people more or fewer opportunities and choices to be physically active.

The characteristics of the built environment that facilitate or constrain physical activity may differ depending on the purpose of the activity. For example, ready access to parks and trails may facilitate walking for exercise; sidewalks and mixed-use development are likely to be more important to encourage walking for local shopping and other utilitarian purposes. The built environment can be changed in ways that increase opportunities for and reduce barriers to physical activity.

The relationship between the built environment and physical activity is complex and operates through many mediating factors, such as sociodemographic characteristics, personal and cultural variables, safety and security, and time allocation. Whether an individual is physically active is determined largely by his or her capacity, propensity, and willingness to make time for physical activity. For example, while public health surveys have found that on average physical activity levels decline with age, many senior citizens remain physically active. Individual behavior is also influenced by the social and physical environment (see Figure ES-1). For example, the social disorder and deteriorated physical condition of many poor inner-city neighborhoods deter physical activity for many residents. These neighborhoods have some of the physical characteristics thought to be conducive to walking and nonmotorized transport—sidewalks, multiple destinations within close proximity, and mixed land uses—and indeed, low-income urban populations report high levels of walking for utilitarian trips. However, they also report low levels of discretionary physical activity. Crime-ridden streets, littered sidewalks, and poorly maintained environments discourage outdoor physical activity other than necessary trips. Time is another mediating factor and is cited by many as a reason for not being more physically active. For some (e.g., single parents, those holding two jobs), making time for physical activity is difficult. For others, particularly those who spend large amounts of leisure time on such sedentary pursuits as watching television, sedentary behavior may reflect the low priority given to physical activity. The role of time has not been well accounted for in examining the relationship between the built environment and physical activity.

The available empirical evidence shows an association between the built environment and physical activity. However, few studies capable of demonstrating a causal relationship have been conducted, and evidence supporting such a relationship is currently sparse. In addition, the characteristics of the built environment most closely associated with physical activity remain to be determined. Preliminary research does provide some evidence suggesting that such factors as access and safety and security are important for some forms of physical activity, such as walking and cycling, and for some population groups. However, the findings are not definitive because it is not known whether these characteristics affect a person's overall level of physical activity or just his or her amount of outdoor walking and cycling. Furthermore, the literature has not established the degree of impact of the built environment and its various characteristics on physical activity levels; the variance by location (e.g., inner city, inner suburb, outer suburb) and population subgroup (e.g., children, the elderly, the disadvantaged); or the importance to total physical activity levels, the primary variable of interest from a public health perspective.

Weaknesses of the current literature include the lack of a sound theoretical framework, inadequate research designs, and incomplete data. The current state of knowledge in this area is limited in part by the lack of a sound theoretical framework to guide empirical work and inadequate research designs. As noted, most of the studies conducted to date have been cross-sectional. Longitudinal study designs using time-series data are also needed to investigate causal relationships between the built environment and physical activity. Studies that distinguish carefully between personal attitudes and choices and external influences on observed behavior are needed to determine how much an observed association between the built environment and physical activity—for example, in an activity-friendly neighborhood—reflects the physical characteristics of the neighborhood versus the lifestyle preferences of those who choose to live there. Appropriate measures of the built environment are still being developed, and efforts to link such measures to travel and health databases are at an early stage.

The built environment in place today has been shaped by long-standing policies and the practices of many decision makers (e.g., policy makers, elected officials, planners, developers, traffic engineers). Many existing development patterns have resulted from zoning and land use ordinances, design guidelines and funding criteria for transportation infrastructure focused primarily on motorized transportation, values and preferences of home owners and home buyers (e.g., suburban lifestyles, single-family housing), and racial and economic concentration of the poor and disinvestment in their neighborhoods. At the same time, the built environment is constantly changing as homes are renovated and new residences, developments, and office complexes are constructed.

CONCLUSIONS

Regular physical activity is important for health, and inadequate physical activity is a major, largely preventable public health problem.

The committee concurs with the strong and well-established scientific evidence linking physical activity to health outcomes and supporting reversal of the decline in overall physical activity levels as a public health priority. The connection between regular physical activity and health, although not the primary focus of this study, has clearly motivated interest in examining the built environment as a potential point of intervention to encourage more active behavior.

Built environments that facilitate more active lifestyles and reduce barriers to physical activity are desirable because of the positive relationship between physical activity and health.

Achieving this goal is challenging in a highly technological society with a built environment that is already in place and often expensive to change. Nevertheless, even small increases in physical activity levels can have important health and economic benefits. Moreover, the built environment is constantly being renovated and rebuilt and new developments are being constructed; these changes provide opportunities to incorporate more activity-conducive environments. In the committee's judgment, such changes would be desirable even in the absence of the goal of increasing physical activity because of their positive social effects on neighborhood safety, sense of community, and quality of life.

Continuing modifications to the built environment provide opportunities, over time, to institute policies and practices that support the provision of more activity-conducive environments.

The long-term decline in physical activity among the U.S. population has been the cumulative result of many changes; thus there are many opportunities for intervention. However, some interventions will be easier to effect than others. For example, formidable hurdles would have to be overcome to substantially modify long-standing policies, such as the current system of zoning regulations and land use controls that reflects the preferences of many suburban home owners and buyers, to allow greater density of development and more mixed land uses. Similarly, many barriers persist to ending concentrations of minority populations and underinvestment in poor neighborhoods and the accompanying social and economic isolation of the poor. More flexible and targeted approaches—context-sensitive design, special overlay districts, traffic calming measures, community policing—have a better chance of gaining support. Construction of new buildings and developments offers promising opportunities for creating more activity-friendly environments. A wider range of such environments should become available as more neotraditional communities[2]

---

[2] *Neotraditional developments* are characterized by land use and street patterns that encourage walking and cycling. These include such features as interconnected street networks, sidewalks, walking and cycling paths, mixed land uses, and higher densities than those of more typical suburban developments. Such communities are also known as new-urbanist developments.

prove financially successful and employers embrace more walking-friendly office complexes to encourage healthier workforces.

Opportunities to increase physical activity levels exist in many settings—at home, at work, at school, in travel, and in leisure. The built environment has the potential to influence physical activity in each of these settings.

Each setting is characterized by different environmental opportunities and constraints that could affect physical activity levels. In some neighborhoods, for example, residents walk for utilitarian purposes. Keeping these neighborhoods safe and providing desirable destinations should help reinforce and perhaps enhance this behavior. In other neighborhoods, walking for utilitarian purposes is limited. In these settings, recreational walking and cycling may offer the greatest potential for increasing physical activity in the daily routine. Of course, individuals can also obtain their daily physical activity by exercising at home. Most Americans spend the majority of their day at home, at work, and at school, and these are important but understudied locations for physical activity, particularly in view of guidelines suggesting that the daily 30-minute minimum of moderate physical activity can be accumulated in many locations and in small (10-minute) time increments.

Many opportunities and potential policies exist for changing the built environment in ways that are more conducive to physical activity, but the available evidence is not sufficient to identify which specific changes would have the most impact on physical activity levels and health outcomes.

Research has not yet identified causal relationships to a point that would enable the committee to provide guidance about cost-beneficial investments or state unequivocally that certain changes to the built environment would lead to more physical activity or be the most efficient ways of increasing such activity. Effective policies to this end are likely to differ for different population groups (e.g., children, youths, the elderly, the disadvantaged), for different purposes of physical activity (e.g., transportation, exercise), and in different contexts (e.g., inner city, inner suburb, outer suburb, rural).

RECOMMENDATIONS

Given the current state of knowledge and the importance of physical activity for health, the committee urges a continuing and well-supported research effort in this area, which Congress should include in its authorization of research funding for health, physical activity, transportation, planning, and other related areas.

Priorities for this research include the following:

- *Interdisciplinary approaches and international collaboration* bringing together the expertise of the public health, physical activity, urban planning, and transportation research communities, among others, both in the United States and abroad.
- *More complete conceptual models* that provide the basis for formulating testable hypotheses, suggesting the variables and relationships for analysis, and interpreting the results.
- *Better research designs,* particularly longitudinal studies that can begin to address causality issues, as well as designs that control more adequately for self-selection bias.
- *More detailed examination and matching of specific characteristics of the built environment with different types of physical activity* to assess the strength of the relationship and the proportion of affected population subgroups. All types of physical activity should be included because there may be substitution among different types. The goal from a public health perspective is an increase in total physical activity levels.

National public health and travel surveys should be expanded to provide more detailed information about the locations of physical activity and travel, which is fundamental to understanding the link between the built environment and physical activity in all contexts.

Geocoding the data on physical activity and health collected in large surveys, such as the Behavioral Risk Factor Surveillance System, the National Health and Nutrition Examination Survey, and the National Health Interview Survey, could help link these rich data sets with information on the built environment and the specific locations where physical activity is occurring. Similarly, travel surveys, such as the National Household Travel Survey, as well as regional travel surveys, should be geocoded to provide more fine-grained geographic detail so researchers can link these surveys and diary data with characteristics of the built environment. In addition, data that reflect a more comprehensive picture of physical activity should be provided. For the public health databases, this means capturing more than leisure-time physical activity; for the travel databases, a more complete accounting should be provided of walking and other forms of nonmotorized travel. More reliable and valid measures of the built environment, both objective and subjective, are also needed. Technologies are available to help verify the accuracy of self-reported data automatically and objectively. Finally, a new database—the Bureau of Labor Statistics' American Time Use Survey—provides an opportunity to track detailed types and durations of respondent activities in many locations. With the collection of extensive demographic and socioeconomic data on the respondents, the database offers researchers a more comprehensive picture of activities and time-use trade-offs by various subgroups of the population than has previously been available. Because the survey is new, opportunities exist to add questions related specifically to physical activity levels.

When changes are made to the built environment—whether retrofitting existing environments or constructing new developments or communities—researchers should view such natural experiments as "demonstration" projects and analyze their impacts on physical activity.

Numerous such opportunities exist, ranging from the construction of new, neotraditional developments to projects of the Active Living by Design program of the Robert Wood Johnson Foundation.[3] To take advantage of these natural experiments, baseline data

---

[3] This program funds projects to develop, implement, and evaluate approaches that support physical activity and promote active living. Partnerships involving local, state, and regional public and nonprofit organizations are eligible and receive grants of up to $200,000 over 5 years.

must be collected. A "rapid-response" capability is needed so that timely funding can be made available to gather the appropriate data when opportunities arise.

Leadership of the Department of Health and Human Services and the Department of Transportation should work collaboratively through an interagency working group to shape an appropriate research agenda and develop a specific recommendation to Congress for a program of research with a defined mission and recommended budget.

An interagency approach is needed because the necessary research does not fall within the purview of any one agency. The committee recognizes that funding for research is currently being provided by the Robert Wood Johnson Foundation and encourages its continuation. Additional funding is needed to enhance research and data collection in several areas and provide a more solid foundation for policy making.

Federally supported research funding should be targeted to high-payoff but difficult-to-finance multiyear projects and enhanced data collection.

The highest priorities, in the committee's judgment, include funding for multiyear longitudinal studies, a rapid-response capability to take advantage of natural experiments as they arise, and support for recommended additions to national databases. The federal government should supplement funding provided by foundations to ensure that this high-payoff research is conducted.

The committee encourages the study of a combined strategy of social marketing and changes to the built environment as interventions to increase physical activity.[4]

The research should be designed to study these approaches both separately and in combination so that the influence of individual

---

[4] Social marketing is the application of commercial marketing techniques to the analysis, planning, execution, and evaluation of programs designed to influence the voluntary behavior of target audiences so as to improve their personal welfare and that of their society.

factors can be evaluated. To be effective, social marketing campaigns should be tailored to different population subgroups with relatively homogeneous characteristics and linked with other interventions involving the built environment for evaluation. For example, a social marketing campaign targeted to low-income, minority populations could be combined with a community policing effort to create safe havens for walking and studied for the effect on increasing physical activity levels in these communities. This more targeted approach should prove more effective than mass messages about the benefits of being physically active. Possible audiences include but are not limited to (*a*) subgroups of the population segmented by gender, age, income, and race; (*b*) public and private officials responsible for community design, development, safety, and public health; (*c*) transportation infrastructure planners and providers; and (*d*) private employers responsible for workplace design and employee information programs and incentives.

Universities should develop interdisciplinary education programs to train professionals in conducting the recommended research and prepare practitioners with appropriate skills at the intersection of physical activity, public health, transportation, and urban planning.

Ideally, new interdisciplinary programs should be developed with a core curriculum that brings together the public health, physical activity, transportation, and urban planning fields in a focused program on the built environment and physical activity. At a minimum, existing programs in public health, transportation, and urban planning should be expanded to provide courses related to physical activity, the built environment, and public health. Similarly, practitioners in the field—local public health workers, physical activity specialists, traffic engineers, and local urban planners—could benefit from supplemental training in these areas.

Those responsible for modifications or additions to the built environment should facilitate access to, enhance the attractiveness of, and ensure the safety and security of places where people can be physically active.

Even though causal connections between the built environment and physical activity levels have not been demonstrated in the literature to date, the available evidence suggests that the built environment can play a facilitating role by providing places and inducements for people to be physically active. Local zoning officials, as well as those responsible for the design and construction of residences, developments, and supporting transportation infrastructure, should be encouraged to provide more activity-friendly environments.

LOOKING FORWARD

The committee believes that research on the relationship between the built environment and physical activity is at a pivotal stage. The number of investigators and studies is growing rapidly; interdisciplinary approaches are being encouraged; and technologies such as the Global Positioning System and geographic information systems, pedometers, and accelerometers are now available to provide and link more objective and detailed measures of both the built environment and physical activity. The committee also recognizes that policy prescriptions require a better understanding of causal connections than currently exists, as well as of the strength of these connections and their impact on population subgroups. In view of the importance of physical activity to health, the committee strongly urges that funding be provided to carry out its recommendations for conducting needed longitudinal studies, evaluating natural experiments, and enhancing data collection. To guide these efforts, the committee recommends a comprehensive approach focused on the individual and social as well as environmental determinants of physically active behavior.

1

Introduction

On the eve of the Centennial Olympic Games held in Atlanta, Georgia, the U.S. Surgeon General released a landmark report on physical activity and health (DHHS 1996). In marked contrast to the fitness and physical achievements of the world's Olympic athletes, the Surgeon General reported that 60 percent of American adults do not meet recommended levels of physical activity,[1] and 25 percent are completely sedentary (DHHS 1996). Sedentary lifestyles are estimated to contribute to as many as 255,000 preventable deaths a year in the United States despite scientific evidence that regular physical activity—even at moderate levels, such as walking briskly for 30 minutes on most days—provides clear health benefits (Hahn et al. 1990 and Powell and Blair 1994 in DHHS 1996).

Concerned about the adverse health effects of physical inactivity, the Robert Wood Johnson Foundation (RWJF) and the Centers for Disease Control and Prevention (CDC) have undertaken environmental health initiatives to explore the causes of Americans' increasingly sedentary lifestyles and identify opportunities to effect change through policies that would encourage greater levels of physical activity. The role of the built environment—in particular, decentralized land use patterns and reliance on the automobile—has come under scrutiny as one important potential contributor to reduced physical activity levels.

---

[1] The experts recommend a minimum of 30 minutes a day of moderate physical activity (e.g., brisk walking) on 5 or more days a week or 20 minutes a day of more vigorous physical activity on 3 or more days a week (DHHS 1996). Historical data on physical activity levels are based on self-reported surveys of leisure-time physical activity only (DHHS 1996).

STUDY CHARGE AND SCOPE

In the above context, this study was requested by RWJF and CDC to examine the role of the built environment in physical activity levels. In particular, this report

- Reviews the broad trends affecting the relationships among physical activity, health, transportation, and land use;
- Summarizes what is known about these relationships and what they suggest for future policy decisions at all levels of government; and
- Identifies priorities for future research.

The built environment is broadly defined to include land use patterns, the transportation system, and design features that together generate needs and provide opportunities for travel and physical activity.[2] It refers to physical environments that have been modified by humans and comprises public spaces, parks, and trails, as well as physical structures (e.g., homes, schools, workplaces) and transportation infrastructure (e.g., streets, sidewalks).

A fairly extensive body of literature exists on the causal relationships between transportation policies and land use, although debate continues about both the direction and strength of those relationships (TRB 1995). Many of the adverse environmental and health effects of low-density development and reliance on automobile travel, such as poor air quality, diminished water supply and quality, and traffic injuries, have also been examined. The present study attempts to extend this understanding to examine the causal role of transportation and land use in increasingly sedentary lifestyles—a connection that has received much less research attention. The study can be viewed as a framing exercise whose objective is to sort out the complex relationships among transportation,

---

[2] *Land use patterns* refers to the spatial distribution of human activities. The *transportation system* refers to the physical infrastructure and services that provide the spatial links or connectivity among activities. *Design* refers to the aesthetic, physical, and functional qualities of the built environment, such as the design of buildings and streetscapes, and relates to both land use patterns and the transportation system (Handy 2004). The reader is directed to the section on definition of key terms in the Handy paper for more details.

land use, physical activity, and health. Are there identifiable characteristics of built environments associated with different levels of physical activity? What are the strength and magnitude of any causal relationships? Do these relations differ by subgroups of the population or by type of physical activity? What implications for policy can be drawn from the current state of knowledge? What methods and data problems must be resolved to improve understanding in this area? What are priorities for future research?

The study is focused primarily on the U.S. experience. International studies and experience are reviewed where relevant. However, differences in land use and travel patterns as well as regulatory and institutional arrangements limit the applicability of foreign experience to the United States.

The remainder of this chapter provides a brief review of the importance of physical activity to health and energy balance, an overview of the committee's approach to the study and key issues considered, and a summary of the organization of the report.

PHYSICAL ACTIVITY AND HEALTH: OVERVIEW

The primary reason for recent interest in the physical activity levels of the U.S. population, both adults and youths, stems from the clear connection between physical activity and health. The Surgeon General's report of 1996 reviewed the existing literature on the role of physical activity in preventing disease. That review revealed an inverse association between physical activity and several diseases that is "moderate in magnitude, consistent across studies that differed substantially in methods and populations, and biologically plausible" (DHHS 1996, 145). The report concluded that the evidence is sufficiently strong to draw a causal relation between physical activity and health outcomes, including reductions in the risk of mortality from all causes, as well as reductions in cardiovascular disease (e.g., heart attacks, strokes), colon cancer, and non-insulin-dependent diabetes. Subsequent research has confirmed that endurance-type physical activity (e.g., walking, cycling) also reduces the risk of developing obesity, osteoporosis, and depression (Saris et al. 2003; Landers and Arent 2001). In addition, physical activity may improve psychological well-being and quality of life (DHHS 1996).

Concern about physical activity levels also stems from economic considerations. According to CDC, direct medical expenses associated with physical inactivity totaled more than $76 billion in 2000 (CDC 2003; Pratt et al. 2000). This figure does not take into account indirect costs, such as lost productivity from the physical and mental disabilities to which sedentary behavior contributes. Research has shown that people who are physically active have, on average, lower annual direct medical costs and fewer hospital stays and physician visits, use fewer medications, miss fewer days of work, and are more productive at work than physically inactive people (Pratt et al. 2000). If 10 percent of adults began walking on a regular basis, an estimated $5.6 billion in heart disease costs alone could be saved (Pratt et al. 2000).

ENERGY BALANCE AND THE OBESITY CONNECTION

An important function of physical activity is to help maintain energy balance. Weight gain occurs when energy intake (calories consumed) exceeds total daily energy expenditure for a prolonged period (DHHS 1996). Total energy expenditure represents the sum of three factors: (*a*) resting energy expenditure to maintain basic body functions (approximately 60 percent of total energy requirements); (*b*) processing of food, which includes the thermic effect of digestion, absorption, transport, and deposition of nutrients (about 10 percent of total energy requirements); and (*c*) nonresting energy expenditure, primarily in the form of physical activity (about 30 percent of total energy requirements) (Leibel et al. 1995 in DHHS 1996). Energy balance tilts to weight gain when disproportionately more energy is taken in. For a typical person, about 1 pound (0.45 kilograms) of fat energy is stored for each 3,500 kilocalories of excess energy intake (DHHS 1996).

Obesity, a major public health problem, is frequently and mistakenly confused with inadequate levels of physical activity—a separate and critical public health problem. The recent marked rise in obesity levels among the U.S. population is due to an energy imbalance. According to the results of a 1999–2000 CDC-sponsored survey, nearly two-thirds of U.S. adults aged 20 and older are overweight or obese,[3] and approximately 15 percent of children and adolescents aged 6 to 19 are overweight (Flegal et al. 2002; Ogden et al. 2002). Among U.S. adults, obesity levels doubled between 1980 and 2000—from 15 percent of the adult population to 31 percent. The percentage of children and adolescents defined as overweight has more than doubled since the early 1970s, with many adverse health consequences (CDC 2004). The 10- to 12-pound median weight gain of the U.S. population over the past two decades is the result of an estimated daily net caloric imbalance of about 100 to 150 calories, equivalent to drinking about two-thirds of a 12-ounce soda each day (Cutler et al. 2003).

Physical activity can play an important role in helping to restore and maintain energy balance. For example, increasing physical activity levels by walking briskly for 1 to 1.5 miles a day (e.g., a 15- or 20-minute mile) could offset the estimated net daily caloric imbalance of 100 to 150 calories (Cutler et al. 2003). Of course, the precise amount of caloric expenditure associated with physical activity is a function of the weight of the individual and the type and duration of the activity (Cutler et al. 2003). In general, however, relatively small changes in physical activity levels can play an important role in weight management and the reversal of obesity trends.

Theories abound concerning the causes of the recent rise in obesity levels—the extent to which it can be attributed to caloric intake

---

[3] Adults are defined as being obese if they have a body mass index (BMI) of 30 or greater, and as being overweight if they have a BMI of 25 but less than 30. Children and adolescents are defined as overweight if they have a BMI above the 95th percentile for their age and sex. A definition of obesity for children and adolescents on the basis of health outcomes or risk factors has not yet been formulated. BMI, one of the most commonly used measures to define overweight and obesity, is calculated as a measure of weight in pounds divided by the square of height in inches, multiplied by 703 (DHHS 2002).

versus caloric expenditure and the role played by physical activity (Cutler et al. 2003). Resolving this debate, however, is not the primary purpose of this study. The focus is on understanding what effects the built environment may have in fostering sedentary behavior, the strength and magnitude of these effects, and opportunities and incentives to encourage greater physical activity.

STUDY APPROACH AND KEY ISSUES

The effects of the built environment on physical activity levels operate through a complex set of relationships. Figure 1-1 shows the committee's conceptualization of the key connections. The starting point is the individual, with all the demographic characteristics, genetic components, lifestyle and other preferences, and time

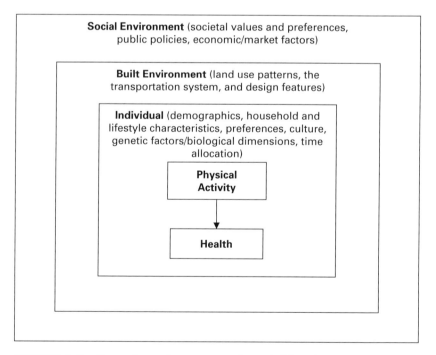

FIGURE 1-1   Overview of conceptual model for the study.

constraints that influence the capacity and propensity to be physically active. For example, some individuals prefer a physically active lifestyle, choose to live in neighborhoods with bicycle lanes and walking trails, and use these and other activity-friendly facilities during their leisure time and, whenever possible, for utilitarian travel. Others are less physically active by choice or are constrained by limited time, income, or physical disabilities.

The figure shows that the individual is embedded in a built environment and in a larger social environment of economic, political, and societal forces that shape the available opportunities and choices for physical activity. For example, those inner-city neighborhoods with high crime rates, boarded-up store fronts, and poorly maintained infrastructure discourage walking or cycling even though the greater accessibility of many destinations, connectivity (directness of travel), and mix of land uses often found in inner cities are important correlates of physical activity (Saelens et al. 2003). Similarly, the character of communities in which individuals live, their daily activity patterns, and their opportunities for physical activity are affected by social norms, such as teenagers' preference for driving to school; government policies, such as those affecting the availability of public transportation; and market forces, such as the demand for low-density living and the high cost of housing, that encourage the development of automobile-dependent communities far from city centers.

Figure 1-2 indicates the primary areas of investigation in this study, namely, the characteristics of the built environment and the various types of physical activity it may influence. Notably, the health box falls outside of this area—not because health is unimportant; indeed, it is the primary reason for the interest in physical activity—but because the link between physical activity and health is well established. As in Figure 1-1, the starting point is the individual, who operates at various geographic scales. The building or site, which has certain characteristics (e.g., stairwells, interior layout, access to and among other structures) that may affect physical activity levels, is the smallest unit of interest. The neighborhood is the next largest geographic unit of interest. It encompasses

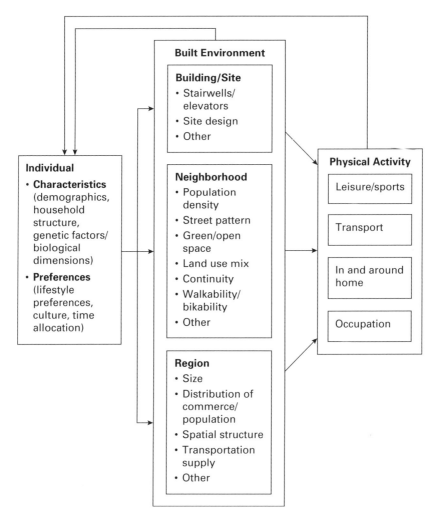

FIGURE 1-2   Detail on areas of interest to this study.

residences, local retail and other commercial services, and schools. Several characteristics of neighborhoods may affect an individual's propensity to be physically active, such as street layout (grid or cul-de-sac); the availability of parks, sidewalks, and bicycle paths; and land use mix (e.g., variety and numbers of destinations). The largest geographic unit for the purposes of this study—the region—is generally defined by the commute area that captures most jobs associated with the resident population. In an urban context, the region is the metropolitan area. Here, the emphasis is on such characteristics as the size of the region, the distribution of jobs and commerce relative to residences, and the supply of transportation facilities (e.g., highways, public transit, bicycle paths) that influence individuals' travel choices and physical activity levels. The focus of this study is primarily on the neighborhood and regional levels; very little is known about physical activity at the building or site level.

Characteristics of the built environment may provide opportunities for the individual to engage in a variety of physical activities. For purposes of this study, physical activity has been categorized into four types (see the rightmost box on Figure 1-2): (*a*) leisure-time recreation and exercise (e.g., bicycle riding, working out at a sports club or on a home treadmill), (*b*) transport or utilitarian travel (e.g., commuting, grocery shopping), (*c*) household production and home maintenance (e.g., housework, gardening, raking leaves), and (*d*) occupation-related physical activity (e.g., physically active jobs, stair climbing at work). The distinctions among these categories, however, are not always clear. For example, walking to run an errand could be counted as both exercise and utilitarian travel.

The diagram illustrates the complexity of the causal chain from the individual to the built environment to physical activity. For example, if a researcher focuses only on the link between the built environment and physical activity, the role of the built environment could be overstated. If, instead, the researcher steps back and controls for individual characteristics, including the possibility that the individual may choose or self-select an activity-friendly environment, the independent effect of the built environment on physical activity may be smaller. The diagram also shows several feedback loops. The built environment may influence the individual (for example, living in a neighborhood in which it is pleasant, safe, and easy to walk to stores may induce a more positive attitude toward utilitarian walking; living in a transit-rich area may increase one's propensity to try transit). Physical activity itself may reinforce the propensity of an individual to be physically active.

An analysis of the linkages between the built environment and physical activity levels raises several key issues. First, scale plays an important role in determining which characteristics of the built environment are likely to affect individual decisions about travel mode and physical activity. For example, such neighborhood characteristics as amount of traffic and availability and proximity of facilities such as sidewalks, local parks, and paths are likely to be important to the decision to walk or cycle in the neighborhood. These characteristics, however, probably have little effect on whether an individual chooses to drive or take transit to work or to a shopping center. That decision is likely to be affected more by relative travel time—a function of distance between origin and destination and proximity and quality of service of available transport modes—as well as trip complexity (e.g., number of destinations, time constraints).

Second, the relationship between the built environment and physical activity operates through many mediating variables. For example, the actual or perceived safety of the environment could affect an individual's propensity to be physically active in certain ways. Safety from crime may be the dominant concern in poor inner-city neighborhoods, while safety from traffic may be the major concern in middle- and higher-income suburban developments. Air quality is another mediating variable. Parents and school officials may limit the outdoor physical activity of school-age children in areas with poor air quality because of adverse health effects. For example, a recent study found that participation in multiple team sports and time spent outside were associated with the development of physician-diagnosed asthma in children of middle-income communities with high concentrations of ozone (McConnell et al. 2002).

Third, the trade-offs individuals make among their travel modes and the kinds of physical activity in which they engage are important in determining total levels of physical activity—the primary dimension of interest from the perspective of energy expenditure and health. For example, an individual may choose to commute to work by car rather than by a more physically active mode, such as bicycling or walking to the bus or subway stop. By using the faster mode, however, that individual may have more time for exercise at a sports club or at home. Alternatively, those who choose to commute by bicycle or transit may forgo other recreational activity once they have reached their destination. Who will have expended the greater level of energy and achieved the greatest health benefits is not readily apparent.

Finally, time is a critical dimension in assessing opportunities for physical activity. Despite the tremendous growth in labor-saving technologies during the past century, particularly in the home, the demands of family, work, and travel limit the time available for physical activity for many individuals, at least during the workweek. Thus, it is important to consider how opportunities for physical activity can be fit into peoples' daily routines at both work and home.

ORGANIZATION OF THE REPORT

The remainder of this report addresses the committee's charge as outlined above. Chapter 2 provides a more complete discussion of the link between physical activity and health and presents data on the current physical activity levels of the U.S. population. In Chapter 3, historical data that may help explain the apparent long-term decline in total physical activity levels are examined in the areas of technological innovations in the workplace, at home, and in travel; decentralization of population and employment; and time use. Chapter 4 explores the contextual factors that affect physical activity levels— from the individual level; to the social context; to the institutional, regulatory, and political forces that have shaped the built environment in place today—and draws implications for intervention. Chapter 5 is concerned with issues in designing research for studying the relationship between the built environment and physical activity, particularly for examining causal connections, while Chapter 6 critically reviews the empirical research and findings to date. In Chapter 7, the committee provides its own findings, conclusions, and recommendations for policy and future research.

REFERENCES

Abbreviations

CDC   Centers for Disease Control and Prevention
DHHS   U.S. Department of Health and Human Services
TRB   Transportation Research Board

CDC. 2003. *Improving Nutrition and Increasing Physical Activity.* www.cdc.gov/nccdphp/bb_nutrition. Accessed Dec. 6, 2003.

CDC. 2004. *Physical Activity.* www.cdc.gov/healthyplaces/healthtopics/physactivity.htm. Accessed Feb. 5, 2004.

Cutler, D. M., E. L. Glaeser, and J. M. Shapiro. 2003. Why Have Americans Become More Obese? *Journal of Economic Perspectives,* Vol. 17, No. 3, Summer, pp. 93–118.

DHHS. 1996. *Physical Activity and Health: A Report of the Surgeon General.* Centers for Disease Control and Prevention, National Center for Chronic Disease Prevention and Health Promotion, Atlanta, Ga.

DHHS. 2002. *Physical Activity Fundamental to Preventing Disease.* aspe.hhs.gov/health/reports/physicalactivity. Accessed Feb. 5, 2004.

Flegal, K. M., M. D. Carroll, C. L. Ogden, and C. L. Johnson. 2002. Prevalence and Trends in Obesity Among U.S. Adults, 1999–2000. *Journal of the American Medical Association,* Vol. 288, pp. 1723–1727.

Hahn, R. A., S. M. Teutsch, R. B. Rothenberg, and J. S. Marks. 1990. Excess Deaths From Nine Chronic Diseases in the United States, 1986. *Journal of the American Medical Association,* Vol. 264, pp. 2654–2659.

Handy, S. 2004. *Critical Assessment of the Literature on the Relationships Among Transportation, Land Use, and Physical Activity.* Department of Environmental Science and Policy, University of California, Davis. Prepared for the Committee on Physical Activity, Health, Transportation, and Land Use, July.

Landers, D. M., and S. M. Arent. 2001. Physical Activity and Mental Health. In *Handbook of Sport Psychology,* 2nd ed. (R. N. Singer, H. A. Hausenblas, and C. M. Janelle, eds.), John Wiley and Sons, New York, pp. 740–765.

Leibel, R. L., M. Rosenbaum, and J. Hirsch. 1995. Changes in Energy Expenditure Resulting from Altered Body Weight. *New England Journal of Medicine,* Vol. 332, pp. 621–628.

McConnell, R., K. Berhane, F. Gilliland, S. J. London. T. Islam, W. J. Gauderman, E. Avoi, H. G. Margolis, and J. M. Peters. 2002. Asthma in Exercising Children Exposed to Ozone: A Cohort Study. *The Lancet,* Vol. 359, pp. 386–391.

Ogden, C. L., K. M. Flegal, M. D. Carroll, and C. L. Johnson. 2002. Prevalence and Trends in Overweight Among U.S. Children and Adolescents, 1999–2000. *Journal of the American Medical Association,* Vol. 288, pp. 1728–1732.

Powell, K. E., and S. N. Blair. 1994. The Public Health Burdens of Sedentary Living Habits: Theoretical but Realistic Estimates. *Medicine and Science in Sports and Exercise,* Vol. 26, pp. 253–287.

Pratt, M., C. A. Macera, and G. Wang. 2000. Higher Direct Medical Costs Associated with Physical Inactivity. *The Physician and Sportsmedicine,* Vol. 28, pp. 63–70.

Saelens, B. E., J. F. Sallis, and L. D. Frank. 2003. Environmental Correlates of Walking and Cycling: Findings from the Transportation, Urban Design, and Planning Literatures. *Annals of Behavioral Medicine,* Vol. 25, No. 2, pp. 80–91.

Saris, W. H. M., S. N. Blair, M. A. van Baak, S. B. Eaton, P. S. W. Davies, L. DiPietro, M. Fogelholm, A. Rissanen, D. Schoeller, B. Swinburn, A. Tremblay, K. R. Westerterp, and H. Wyatt. 2003. How Much Physical Activity Is Enough to Prevent Unhealthy Weight Gain? Outcome of the IASO 1st Stock Conference and Consensus Statement. *Obesity Reviews,* Vol. 4, pp. 101–114.

TRB. 1995. *Special Report 245: Expanding Metropolitan Highways: Implications for Air Quality and Energy Use.* National Research Council, Washington, D.C.

SUMMARY

Physical Activity and Health

The evidence provided in this chapter demonstrates a strong and well-established scientific basis for linking physical activity to health outcomes. Current guidelines recommend either vigorous-intensity activity for at least 20 minutes per day for a minimum of 3 days a week or moderate-intensity activity for at least 30 minutes per day on all (or a minimum of 5) days of the week. The latter activity can accumulate over the course of a day in sessions of at least 10 minutes. Yet current survey data indicate that the majority of the U.S. population falls short of achieving these targets. More than half of adults report not meeting recommended levels of physical activity, and more than one-quarter characterize themselves as being completely inactive during their leisure time. Nearly one-third of high-school-age teenagers report not meeting recommended levels of physical activity, and 10 percent classify themselves as inactive. Approximately half are enrolled in a physical education class, but only one-third attend such classes daily. More than two-fifths of younger children, aged 9 to 13, report not participating in organized physical activity outside of school; slightly less than one-quarter indicate that they do not participate in any free-time physical activity during nonschool hours. These results indicate a widespread but largely preventable public health problem whose causes and possible solutions present a challenge to understand.

In the next chapter, longitudinal data are analyzed to determine what is known about changes in physical activity levels over time and the direction of these changes. Trends in other areas, including land use patterns and travel behavior—the focus of this study—are examined for their possible contribution to these changes.

2
Physical Activity and Health

Drawing on the Surgeon General's 1996 report (DHHS 1996) and subsequent research, this chapter briefly summarizes the state of knowledge about the effects of physical activity on health, as well as recommendations on physical activity levels for adults and for children and adolescents. Methods and data for monitoring physical activity levels are then discussed, and current results for the U.S. population are compared with the recommended levels.

TERMINOLOGY

The terms *physical activity, physical fitness,* and *exercise* are often used interchangeably but have distinct meanings:

- Physical activity can be defined as "bodily movement produced by the contraction of skeletal muscle that increases energy expenditure above the basal level" (DHHS 1996, 20). It is often categorized by the context in which it occurs, such as leisure time, transport, household, and occupation (see Figure 1-2 in Chapter 1).
- Physical fitness can be defined as the "ability to carry out daily tasks with vigor and alertness, without undue fatigue, and with ample energy to enjoy leisure-time pursuits and to meet unforeseen emergencies" (Park 1989). Attributes of physical fitness include cardiorespiratory endurance; flexibility; balance; body composition; and muscular endurance, strength, and power. The term can be used to describe either athletic- and performance-

related fitness or health-related fitness (DHHS 1996). Depending on the individual's performance or health goal, specific attributes of physical fitness become more important (Caspersen et al. 1985; Pate 1983). For example, achieving a certain level of cardio-respiratory fitness—a health-related fitness goal—requires an increase in cardiorespiratory endurance that can either help reduce the risk of cardiovascular disease or improve the life and overall health of a person who already has the disease.

- Exercise is considered a subcategory of physical activity and has been defined as "physical activity that is planned, structured, repetitive, and purposive in the sense that improvement or maintenance of one or more components of physical fitness is the objective" (Caspersen et al. 1985).

This study uses the broadest possible definition of physical activity because all types of such activity contribute to health. Health is broadly defined as a "state of complete physical, mental, and social well-being and not merely the absence of disease or infirmity" (WHO 1946). Total activity levels—purposeful physical activity or exercise, as well as utilitarian physical activity that occurs in the home, at work, and in travel—are of interest.

EFFECTS OF PHYSICAL ACTIVITY ON HEALTH

The Science Base

The Surgeon General's 1996 report (DHHS 1996) examined the results of hundreds of research studies on the effects of physical activity on health from such fields as epidemiology, exercise physiology, medicine, and the behavioral sciences. The research was focused primarily on endurance-type physical activity, that is, on activity that involves repetitive use of large muscle groups, such as those used in walking and cycling.

Observational or epidemiologic studies have been conducted to determine health effects by comparing the activity levels of individuals who develop specific diseases or health conditions and those who do not. Epidemiologic studies include cohort, case-control, and cross-sectional research designed to estimate the relative magnitude or strength of an association between physical activity or cardiorespiratory fitness levels and a specific health outcome. Cohort studies follow a population to observe how physical activity levels or habits affect the incidence of disease or mortality. In contrast, case-control studies start with a group of individuals (the case group) with a specific disease or health condition of interest, who are then asked to recall their previous level and intensity of physical activity. Their previous level of physical activity is compared with that of a control group that does not have the disease or health condition of interest. Cross-sectional studies assess the association between physical activity and disease at the same point in time; thus they offer limited ability to draw causal inferences between the two variables.

Clinical trials, in comparison, assess the relationship between health outcomes and physical activity by experimentally altering the activity patterns, levels, and intensities within a relatively controlled environment, such as in a laboratory or an exercise program (DHHS 1996). Often considered the gold standard of studies, clinical trials are extremely expensive and time-consuming and require that every precaution be taken to protect the study participants. The high cost and feasibility constraints of large-scale clinical trials have thus far prohibited such designs with major morbidity or mortality as health outcomes. Instead, the effect of physical activity on intermediate outcomes, such as fitness or coronary heart disease risk factors, has been evaluated.

Most studies reviewed in the Surgeon General's 1996 report were cohort studies; that is, they assessed whether an association existed between some baseline level of physical activity or fitness and the development of specific health outcomes. The majority of the studies controlled for important confounding factors that might have biased the results, such as age, body weight, smoking, blood pressure, blood lipid levels, alcohol consumption, and disease status. Numerous studies were analyzed to determine (*a*) the consistency across studies of an association between physical activity and disease incidence; (*b*) the magnitude or strength of the association; (*c*) whether there was evidence that the level of activity preceded the development of disease; (*d*) the presence of a dose-response relationship, that is, whether higher amounts of physical activity conferred greater health benefits; and (*e*) the biological plausibility of the relationship, that is, the underlying physiological mechanisms that can explain why physical activity has a protective or restorative effect on specific health outcomes.

Benefits of Physical Activity

The Surgeon General's report concluded that physical activity is causally related to health outcomes. It cited convincing and biologically plausible evidence of consistent and strong inverse relationships between physical activity or fitness and numerous diseases. For most health conditions, longitudinal data confirmed the temporal effects of regular physical activity on disease reduction. Moreover, increasing amounts of physical activity were associated with decreasing risk of disease.

Both older and younger adults who exercise regularly or lead a physically active lifestyle have lower mortality rates and live longer than those who are physically inactive (Kaplan et al. 1996; Paffenbarger et al. 1993; Sherman et al. 1994). More specifically, even in the absence of controlled clinical trials, there is sufficient evidence that regular physical activity reduces the risk of developing or dying from several of the leading chronic diseases in the United States (see Box 2-1). For example, the 1996 report found that regular physical activity or cardiorespiratory fitness reduces the risk of dying from coronary heart disease. The strength of the association is similar in magnitude to that of the relationship between coronary heart disease and smoking, hypertension, or elevated cholesterol. Moreover, the report found that regular physical activity prevents or delays the development of high blood pressure—a risk factor for coronary heart disease—and reduces blood pressure in those who already exhibit hypertension.

BOX 2-1

Health Benefits of Regular Physical Activity

- Reduces the risk of dying prematurely from cardiovascular diseases, such as coronary heart disease and stroke.
- Reduces the risk of developing non-insulin-dependent diabetes.
- Reduces the risk of developing high blood pressure or hypertension.
- Reduces blood pressure in those already with hypertension.
- Reduces the risk of developing colon cancer.
- Reduces the risk of developing breast cancer (Vainio and Bianchini 2002).
- Reduces the development of osteoarthritis and osteoporosis.
- Reduces fall-related injuries among older adults.
- Helps maintain a healthy weight and reduce overweight and obesity.
- Helps build and maintain healthy bones, muscles, and joints.
- Reduces feelings of depression and anxiety and promotes physiological well-being.

SOURCES: DHHS 1996; DHHS 2002.

The benefits of regular physical activity to both the individual and society are compelling. Currently, chronic diseases account for 7 of every 10 deaths in the United States and more than 60 percent of all medical expenditures (CDC 2003b). Every year, as many as 255,000 U.S. adults die from causes that may be attributed to physical inactivity alone and 300,000 from inactivity and poor diet combined; these figures do not include others who suffer from chronic disease and impaired quality of life (Hahn et al. 1990; Powell and Blair 1994; McGinnis and Foege 1993). According to another estimate, 32 to 35 percent of all deaths in the United States attributable to coronary heart disease, colon cancer, and diabetes could be prevented if all members of the population were physically active (Powell and Blair 1994).

The benefits of physical activity appear to extend to all segments of the population. For example, even seniors and those with disabilities and chronic disease conditions benefit from physical activity, which improves their mobility and physical, mental, and social functioning (Butler et al. 1998). Regular participation in physical activity during childhood and adolescence helps build and maintain healthy bones, muscles, and joints; helps control weight, build muscle, and reduce fat; prevents or delays the development of high blood pressure and helps reduce blood pressure in adolescents with hypertension; and reduces feelings of depression and anxiety (DHHS 1996; Report to the President 2000). Indeed, more recent research supports stronger conclusions than those presented in the Surgeon General's 1996 report on the effect of physical activity on mental health (Landers and Arent 2001).[1]

Although additional studies are needed to demonstrate a conclusive relationship between being physically active as a child and adolescent and achieving higher levels of academic performance, several studies are suggestive in this regard (Pate et al. 1996; Sallis et al. 1999). Participation in physical activity among adolescents has been shown to increase self-esteem, reduce anxiety and stress, and promote a sense of social well-being. Adolescents who participate in interscholastic sports are less likely to be regular or heavy smokers or drug users and to engage in violent behavior, and they are more likely to stay in school and have good conduct and high academic achievement (Escobedo et al. 1993; Pate et al. 1996; Zill et al. 1995).

RECOMMENDED LEVELS OF PHYSICAL ACTIVITY

The direct causal relationship between physical activity and health benefits raises questions about the type and amount of activity needed to produce those benefits. Physical activity regimens can

---

[1] A meta-analysis of relevant research found that the overall magnitude of the effects of exercise on anxiety, depression, stress, and cognitive functioning ranges from small to moderate, but in all cases, these effects are statistically significant (Landers and Arent 2001).

be designed to meet any individual's needs, desires, and capacities; however, the primary focus at the national level has been on developing recommendations to help broad segments of the population achieve health benefits. Since the mid-1960s the available scientific evidence has been used as the basis for recommendations on physical activity that vary in their objective (e.g., sports performance, overall health promotion, weight maintenance or loss, disease-specific prevention); type of activity (e.g., endurance, strength, flexibility training); and the activity's intensity (i.e., rate of energy expenditure), frequency (e.g., number of sessions engaged in over a week), and duration (i.e., length of time spent being physically active) (Bouchard and Shephard 1994; DHHS 1996).

Adults

In 1980, the U.S. Department of Health and Human Services (DHHS) stated that adults can achieve significant health benefits from participating in vigorous-intensity activity for at least 20 minutes per day for a minimum of 3 days a week (DHHS 1980).[2] Vigorous-intensity activities are defined as those that raise the rate of energy expenditure, expressed as metabolic equivalents (METs), more than sixfold above resting levels.[3] Assuming that 1 MET is equivalent to 1 kilocalorie per kilogram body weight per hour, jogging at a 7 MET level burns approximately 7 kilocalories per minute (kcal/min) for a person weighing 60 kilograms (132 pounds). A healthy individual might also burn 7 kcal/min while engaging in heavy yard work, participating in an aerobics class, swimming continuous laps, or bicycling vigorously (Ainsworth et al. 2000).

Over the next decade, epidemiologic evidence not only continued to provide strong evidence of the relationship between physical activity and health but also revealed that substantial benefits

---

[2] The DHHS recommendations were based on an earlier position paper by the American College of Sports Medicine recommending both the quantity and quality of exercise needed to develop and maintain fitness in healthy adults (ACSM 1978).

[3] MET is defined as the ratio of the working metabolic rate to the resting metabolic rate (Ainsworth et al. 2000).

accrue from even moderate amounts and types of activity.[4] As a result, the Centers for Disease Control and Prevention (CDC) and the American College of Sports Medicine (ACSM) released a joint statement in 1995—rearticulated in the Surgeon General's 1996 report—that most adults will achieve substantial health benefits if they accumulate a minimum of 30 minutes of moderate-intensity activity preferably on all days of the week (at least 5 days a week minimum) (Pate et al. 1995).[5] Moderate-intensity activity is defined as any activity that raises the rate of energy expenditure three to six times above resting levels (3 to 6 METs). For a 60-kilogram person, activity at these levels burns 3 to 6 kcal/min—an amount a healthy person would burn while walking briskly, mowing the lawn, dancing, swimming for recreation, or bicycling (Ainsworth et al. 2000). The evidence available at the time suggested that this activity could be accumulated over the course of a day in sessions of at least 10 minutes, rather than having to be performed in one longer continuous session, although it was noted that more research was needed on the relative health benefits. It was clear, however, that intermittent episodes of activity are more beneficial than being sedentary (DHHS 1996).

The Surgeon General's 1996 report acknowledged that for most people, greater health benefits can be obtained by engaging in physical activity of more vigorous intensity or of longer duration than the

---

[4] In fact, it has been shown that physical activity is related to health outcomes in a dose-response fashion, such that the amount of benefit is proportional to the amount of physical activity; there is no threshold level of activity necessary before health benefits accrue (DHHS 1996). Nevertheless, some studies that have quantified the amount of physical activity associated with improved health outcomes have found that certain levels of kilocalorie energy expenditure from physical activity are associated with different levels of reduction in the risk of mortality and morbidity (Paffenbarger et al. 1986; Leon et al. 1987; Slattery et al. 1989; Helmrich et al. 1991). These studies provided the basis for the finding that a minimum increase in daily energy expenditure of approximately 150 kilocalories per day is associated with substantial health benefits, which can be achieved by moderate levels of physical activity, such as walking briskly for 30 minutes per day (DHHS 1996).

[5] Special physical activity recommendations exist for seniors and those with disabilities and certain illnesses who want to increase their level of physical activity and achieve the associated health advantages. Additional information on recommendations for these populations can be found on CDC's website at www.cdc.gov/nccdphp/dnpa/physical/recommendations.

30-minute minimum. Evidence from more recent epidemiological, observational, and intervention studies confirms this finding (Manson et al. 2002; Myers et al. 2002; Kraus et al. 2002), although the optimal amount of physical activity to achieve health benefits has not been established and probably varies from person to person.[6]

Children and Adolescents

The National Association for Sport and Physical Education recommends that children in elementary school accumulate at least 30 to 60 minutes of age- and developmentally appropriate physical activity from a variety of activities on all or most days of the week (NASPE Council on Physical Education for Children 2004). The activity should vary between moderate and vigorous intensity, with appropriate periods of rest and recovery to prevent injury. Children should avoid extended periods of inactivity.

In 1994, the International Consensus Conference on Physical Activity Guidelines for Adolescents recommended that adolescents be physically active daily or nearly every day as part of play, games, sports, work, transportation, recreation, physical education, or planned exercise in the context of family, school, and community activities. Adolescents should engage in three or more sessions per week of activities that last 20 minutes or more at a time and require moderate to vigorous levels of exertion.

National Health Goals

In addition to physical activity guidelines, the federal government has periodically set physical activity goals for the nation for both adults and adolescents. The recent national prevention agenda *Healthy People 2010* sets forth various objectives designed to reduce the most significant preventable threats to health (DHHS 2000). The objectives related to physical activity are listed in Box 2-2.

In addition to setting these goals, *Healthy People 2010* established physical activity as one of 10 leading health indicators (Box 2-3)

---

[6] The Institute of Medicine has reported that physical activity closer to 60 minutes per day provides additional health benefits and helps maintain a healthy body weight (IOM 2002).

BOX 2-2

Healthy People 2010's National Objectives
for Physical Activity

- Reduce the proportion of adults who engage in no leisure-time physical activity to 20 percent or lower.
- Increase the proportion of adults who engage in regular, preferably daily, moderate levels of physical activity for at least 30 minutes a day to 30 percent or more.
- Increase the proportion of adults who engage in vigorous levels of physical activity on 3 or more days per week for at least 20 minutes to 30 percent or more.
- Increase the proportion of adolescents who engage in moderate physical activity for at least 30 minutes on 5 or more days a week.
- Increase the proportion of adolescents who engage in vigorous physical activity that promotes cardiovascular fitness on 3 or more days a week for 20 or more minutes per occasion.
- Increase the proportion of public and private schools that require daily physical education classes and decrease the proportion of adolescents who watch more than 2 hours of television on a school day.
- Increase the proportion of trips of 1 mile or less made by walking to 25 percent of trips among adults and 50 percent among children and adolescents.[a]
- Increase the proportion of trips of 5 miles or less by bicycling to 2 percent of trips among adults and of trips to school of 2 miles or less to 5 percent among children and adolescents.[a]

[a] Baseline data came from the 1995 Nationwide Personal Transportation Survey of the U.S. Department of Transportation.
SOURCE: DHHS 2000.

BOX 2-3

Healthy People 2010's Leading Health Indicators

- Physical activity
- Overweight and obesity
- Tobacco use
- Substance abuse
- Responsible sexual behavior
- Mental health
- Injury and violence
- Environmental quality
- Immunization
- Access to care

SOURCE: DHHS 2000.

that will be used to measure the overall health of the nation. In fact, physical activity is listed first, followed by overweight and obesity and tobacco use, respectively. These represent the major public health issues facing the nation and areas in which improvements can have a significant impact on the health of the American population (DHHS 2000).[7]

MEASURING PHYSICAL ACTIVITY

The ability to demonstrate a relationship between physical activity and health benefits is dependent on measures of physical activity and specific health outcomes that are accurate, precise, and reproducible (NCHS 1989; Wilson et al. 1986). Although limitations still exist, such as the fact that vigorous activities are reported more accurately than moderate or light ones, measures of physical activity have improved over time (Ainsworth et al. 1994; DHHS 1996).

---

[7] The leading indicators were chosen on the basis of their ability to motivate action, the availability of data to measure progress, and their relevance as broad public health issues (DHHS 2000).

Measurement Techniques

Today, most research on physical activity levels relies on (*a*) self-reports, such as diaries, logs, and recall surveys; (*b*) direct monitoring through behavioral observations or mechanical or electronic devices; or (*c*) indirect measures, such as those of cardiorespiratory fitness based on exercise test tolerance, maximal oxygen uptake, or aerobic power.

Although self-reported measures of physical activity, such as surveys, are subject to recall bias and nonrepresentative sampling of activity depending on the time period about which they inquire, they are relatively easy to administer, inexpensive, and acceptable to study participants. The simplest form of self-reported information about physical activity allows subjects to be placed in hierarchical categories, such as "more or less active than their peers" or "numbers of days on which they were active in the past week." More complex self-reported information about the frequency, duration, and intensity of physical activities can be converted into estimates of energy expenditure in terms of kilocalories, kilojoules, or METs. Responses are often classified according to an external standard, such as how well subjects meet physical activity recommendations.[8]

Direct monitoring eliminates many of the limitations associated with self-reported measures. However, it is expensive, time-consuming, and burdensome to study participants, surveyors, or both. As a result, self-reported measures of physical activity have been used more commonly in assessing the relationship between activity and health (DHHS 1996).[9] As technology advances, objective monitoring is becoming increasingly available for large-scale

---

[8] Typically, survey respondents are classified into three levels: (*a*) sufficiently active (meet physical activity recommendations), (*b*) insufficiently active (some reported physical activity, but not enough to meet existing recommendations), and (*c*) inactive (no reported physical activity) (CDC 2003a).

[9] Because self-reported levels of physical activity tend to be overstated, the fact that such data show an inverse relationship for morbidity and mortality further strengthens the causal inference. Studies on cardiorespiratory fitness—an objective laboratory measure—generally show a stronger association than self-reported physical activity measures for numerous health outcomes (Lee et al. 1999; Wei et al. 1999).

studies, although validity and reliability issues remain (Granner and Sharpe 2004). Measurement issues are discussed in detail in Chapter 5.

Databases

Patterns of physical activity in the United States can be gleaned from several national surveys, including the Behavioral Risk Factor Surveillance System (BRFSS), the National Health Interview Survey (NHIS), the National Health and Nutrition Examination Survey (NHANES), the Youth Risk Behavior Survey System (YRBSS), and the National Household Travel Survey (NHTS) (see Table 2-1). Each provides a part of the picture of the activity levels of Americans by different age groups, ethnicities, education and income levels, and geographic locations. Although each survey has its own purpose and uses different questions to inquire about levels of physical activity and inactivity, collectively their results demonstrate that Americans overall are not achieving the recommended levels (CDC 2003a). The primary databases used in this study to examine current levels and trends in physical activity are described below. A more complete discussion of all the relevant databases can be found in the papers by Brownson and Boehmer (2004) and Boarnet (2004) commissioned by the committee.

Two databases in particular provide current and trend data on the extent to which the U.S. population is meeting recommended physical activity guidelines. Begun in 1984, the CDC-coordinated BRFSS is the leading database for both current and longitudinal data on physical activity levels among U.S. adults. Its aim is to track major behavioral health risk factors, such as physical inactivity. Self-reported telephone interviews are used to derive estimates of how many adult Americans meet recommended physical activity levels (either the vigorous-intensity or moderate-intensity activity level recommendations put forward by DHHS, CDC, and ACSM), how many are insufficiently active, and how many are inactive or sedentary.

The strengths of the survey are its sample size, provision of state- and in some cases city-specific data, ability to estimate physical

TABLE 2-1 Data Sources for Trend Analysis of U.S. Physical Activity Levels

Survey	Mode of Data Collection	Target Population	Frequency of Data Collection	Type of Physical Activity	Purpose
BRFSS	Telephone interview	Adults (≥18 years of age) in U.S. states, territories, and the District of Columbia—approximately 210,000 respondents in 2001	Ongoing—annual	Vigorous, moderate	To provide ongoing statistics on major behavioral risk factors among American adults, including tracking the proportion of respondents who meet recommendations for physical activity levels.
NHIS	Personal interview	Adults and children in U.S. states and the District of Columbia—approximately 100,000 respondents in 2001	Ongoing—annual	Leisure-time Daily activity (i.e., non-leisure-time)	To track progress toward meeting national health objectives.
NHANES	Interview/examination	Children and adults in United States—approximately 10,000 respondents in 1999–2000	Ongoing—annual	Leisure-time (adults), domestic (adults), transport (adults); leisure-time (children)	To provide statistics on dietary intake, nutrition, and health outcomes; physical activity questions first asked in 1999. Only national data on physical fitness measures in adults.
YRBSS	Pencil/paper survey completed at school	U.S. high school students—more than 15,000 respondents in 2000	Every 2 years	Vigorous, moderate, school PE, television watching	To determine national prevalence and age at initiation of key health risk behaviors.
NHTS	Household survey	U.S. households—more than 25,000 respondents in 2001	Every 5 to 7 years	Transportation	To provide national estimates of daily trip frequency, trip distance, means of transportation, and trip time.

NOTE: BRFSS = Behavioral Risk Factor Surveillance System; NHANES = National Health and Nutrition Examination Survey; NHIS = National Health Interview Survey; NHTS = National Household Travel Survey; PE = physical education; YRBSS = Youth Risk Behavior Survey System.
SOURCES: CDC 2003c; NCHS 2003.

activity for subgroups (e.g., women, ethnic groups), and relative consistency of questions over time. Its weaknesses include reliance on self-reported data, lack of coverage for some population subgroups (e.g., low-income individuals who may not have a telephone), and, until 2001, its focus on leisure-time physical activity only. In 2001, survey questions were modified to encompass three types of physical activity—leisure-time, domestic, and transportation.[10] A fourth type of physical activity—occupational—is also captured in the BRFSS. Because of technical issues, however, self-reported occupational activity does not contribute to the overall physical activity score for each individual responding to the survey (CDC 2003a). As a result of the changes in 2001, moreover, estimates based on that survey are not comparable with the estimates from 1984 to 2000.[11]

The YRBSS was developed in 1990 to help determine the onset and national prevalence of key risk behaviors that contribute to death, disability, and social problems among U.S. youth. Conducted biennially, the YRBSS is a national school-based survey of representative samples of students in 9th through 12th grades. Self-reported survey data relevant to physical activity levels among youth include estimates of participation in daily physical education classes and the percentage meeting recommended standards for physical activity. The strength of the survey is its focus on youth as an important population group and oversampling in some cities to allow comparisons by geographic setting. Its limitations include reliance on self-reported data, school-based administration of the survey, and more limited longitudinal data than the BRFSS.

---

[10] Survey respondents were asked whether in the past month they had participated in any physical activities or exercise, such as running, calisthenics, golf, gardening, or walking for exercise. These activities were understood to be forms of leisure-time physical activity. In 2001, the phrase "other than your regular job" was added for clarification (Ham et al. 2004, 83).

[11] The NHIS, used to track the nation's progress against national health goals, also relies on personal interviews for data collection. Before 2000, levels of leisure-time physical activity only were assessed. In 2000, questions concerning usual daily activities related to moving about (e.g., walking, standing, sitting) and lifting and carrying were included to assess the level of physical activity during nonleisure times (CDC 2003a; NCHS 2003).

CDC recently launched a new national telephone survey—the Youth Media Campaign Longitudinal Survey (YMCLS)—of children aged 9 to 13 and their parents. The purpose is to obtain data on physical activity levels among children of this age group. Children are asked about their participation in physical activity during nonschool hours, and parents are asked about perceived barriers to their children's engaging in physical activity.

The NHTS, which combines two former surveys—the Nationwide Personal Transportation Survey and the American Travel Survey—is conducted by the U.S. Department of Transportation to provide data on both the short- and long-term travel behavior of the U.S. population. Conducted every 5 to 7 years, it draws on a nationally representative sample of households and uses travel diaries to derive national estimates of travel type, frequency, mode, and time. These data are the primary source of information on physical activity, particularly walking and bicycling, associated with transportation. Longitudinal data going back as far as 1969 are available for some characteristics. Data on nonmotorized travel (walking and bicycling) have improved in recent years. For example, the most recent survey (2001) gathered additional such data, particularly for walking trips (e.g., trips for walking the dog were to be included in the travel diaries). At the same time, however, the results are not comparable with earlier data.

CURRENT LEVELS OF PHYSICAL ACTIVITY

Results from the 2001 BRFSS indicate that, even with a more complete measure of physical activity than that previously used, fewer than half of all U.S. adults engage in enough physical activity to meet the public health recommendations cited earlier (i.e., at least 30 minutes of moderate-intensity activity per day for at least 5 days a week or at least 20 minutes of vigorous-intensity activity per day for at least 3 days a week) (see Table 2-2). Approximately one-quarter of all U.S. adults reported being completely inactive during their leisure

TABLE 2-2   Summary Statistics on Current Physical Activity Levels Compared with Recommended Guidelines, U.S. Adults and Adolescents

Population	Data Source	Percent Not Meeting Recommended Guidelines	Percent Inactive
Adults (18 years or older)	BRFSS 2001	55	26
Adolescents (9th to 12th grade)	YRBSS 2001	31	10

NOTE: BRFSS = Behavioral Risk Factor Surveillance System; YRBSS = Youth Risk Behavior Survey System.
SOURCES: CDC 2002; CDC 2003d.

time (CDC 2003d).[12] The data show that activity levels decrease with age and are lower among women, ethnic and racial minorities, those with less education and low income levels, the disabled, and those living in the southeastern region of the nation (CDC 2003d).

Insufficient levels of physical activity are not limited to adults. The YRBSS for 2001 revealed that nationwide, nearly one-third of students enrolled in 9th through 12th grades engaged in insufficient amounts of physical activity relative to recommended levels (i.e., had not participated in vigorous physical activity for 20 minutes or more at least three times in the week preceding the survey, or in moderate physical activity for 30 minutes or more at least five times in that week) (CDC 2002) (see Table 2-2). Nearly 10 percent characterized themselves as inactive; that is, they reported not participating in either vigorous or moderate physical activity in the week preceding the survey. Levels of inactivity were higher for female and minority students and increased for all students by grade level (CDC 2002). Nationwide, 52 percent of students were enrolled in a physical education class, but only about one-third attended such a class daily. Approximately 55 percent of students indicated that

---

[12] The 2000 BRFSS, which, as noted, used a less complete measure of physical activity than the 2001 survey, found that only 26 percent of U.S. adults met the recommended physical activity levels, and 27 percent were completely inactive (CDC 2003d). Walking was listed as the primary form of physical activity.

they had played on one or more sports teams during the 12 months preceding the survey. Levels of television watching were high; nearly two-fifths of students reported that they had watched television 3 or more hours on an average school day (CDC 2002).

The 2002 baseline assessment of the YMCLS found that 62 percent of U.S. children aged 9 to 13 did not participate in any organized physical activity during their nonschool hours, and 23 percent did not take part in any physical activity during their free time (CDC 2003c). Significantly lower levels of regular nonschool physical activity were found among non-Hispanic black and Hispanic children and children with parents who had lower incomes and educational levels (CDC 2003c). Parents of all races, incomes, and educational levels perceived many of the same barriers to their children's participating in physical activities. However, transportation difficulties, lack of area opportunities, and expense were reported significantly more often by non-Hispanic black and Hispanic parents than by non-Hispanic white parents. Concerns about neighborhood safety were greater for Hispanic than for non-Hispanic white or black parents (CDC 2003c). Summary data on physical activity levels for younger children are not available.[13]

Results from the 2001 NHTS, the primary source of data on physical activity for travel,[14] showed, not surprisingly, that the vast majority of daily trips (87 percent) were taken by personal vehicle (BTS 2003). Walking, however, accounted for the next highest percentage—almost 9 percent of all trips. Cycling accounted for less than 1 percent of all trips, while trips by transit, including school bus—which involve some walking to reach the transit or bus line—represented slightly more than 3 percent of all trips (2001 NHTS trip results). Because walking and cycling are more prevalent on shorter trips, the NHTS also asked about travel mode for such trips. Adults (those at least 18 years of age) reported walking on 27 percent of

---

[13] A major challenge is how to measure physical activity in younger children without intruding into their normal daily routines. As suggested above, surveys of parents and children face recall problems (IOM 2004).

[14] Travel for recreational purposes is included, so there is some overlap with leisure-time physical activity.

trips of 1 mile or less and cycling on 0.6 percent of trips of 5 miles or less (2001 NHTS special data runs). Children aged 5 to 15 reported walking on 36 percent of school trips of 1 mile or less and cycling on 1.5 percent of school trips of 2 miles or less (2001 NHTS special data runs).

REFERENCES

Abbreviations

ACSM	American College of Sports Medicine
BTS	Bureau of Transportation Statistics
CDC	Centers for Disease Control and Prevention
DHHS	U.S. Department of Health and Human Services
IOM	Institute of Medicine
NASPE	National Association for Sport and Physical Education
NCHS	National Center for Health Statistics
WHO	World Health Organization

ACSM. 1978. The Recommended Quantity and Quality of Exercise for Developing and Maintaining Fitness in Healthy Adults. *Medicine and Science in Sports,* Vol. 10, pp. vii–xi.

Ainsworth, B. E., W. L. Haskell, M. C. Whitt, M. L. Irwin, A. M. Swartz, S. J. Strath, W. L. O'Brien, D. R. Bassett, Jr., K. H. Schmitz, P. O. Emplaincourt, D. R. Jacobs, Jr., and A. S. Leon. 2000. Compendium of Physical Activities: An Update of Physical Activity Codes and MET Intensities. *Medicine and Science in Sports and Exercise,* Vol. 32, No. 9 (Supplement), pp. S498–S504.

Ainsworth, B. E., H. J. Montoye, and A. S. Leon. 1994. Methods of Assessing Physical Activity During Leisure and Work. In *Physical Activity, Fitness, and Health: International Proceedings and Consensus Statement* (C. Bouchard, R. J. Shephard, and T. Stephens, eds.), Human Kinetics, Champaign, Ill., pp. 146–159.

Boarnet, M. G. 2004. *The Built Environment and Physical Activity: Empirical Methods and Data Resources.* University of California, Irvine. Prepared for the Committee on Physical Activity, Health, Transportation, and Land Use, July 18.

Bouchard, C., and R. J. Shephard. 1994. Physical Activity, Fitness, and Health: The Model and Key Concepts. In *Physical Activity, Fitness, and Health: International Proceedings and Consensus Statement* (C. Bouchard, R. J. Shephard, and J. Stephens, eds.), Human Kinetics, Champaign, Ill.

Brownson, R. C., and T. K. Boehmer. 2004. *Patterns and Trends in Physical Activity, Occupation, Transportation, Land Use, and Sedentary Behaviors.* School of Public Health,

St. Louis University. Prepared for the Committee on Physical Activity, Health, Transportation, and Land Use, June 25.

BTS. 2003. *NHTS 2001 Highlight Report.* BTS03-05. U.S. Department of Transportation.

Butler, R. N., R. Davis, C. B. Lewis, M. E. Nelson, and E. Strauss. 1998. Physical Fitness: Benefits of Exercise for the Older Patient. *Geriatrics,* Vol. 53, No. 10, pp. 46–62.

Caspersen, C. J., K. E. Powell, and G. M. Christensen. 1985. Physical Activity, Exercise, and Physical Fitness: Definitions and Distinctions for Health-Related Research. *Public Health Reports,* Vol. 100, pp. 126–131.

CDC. 2002. Youth Risk Behavior Surveillance—United States, 2001. *Morbidity and Mortality Weekly Report Surveillance Summaries,* Vol. 51, No. SS-4, June 28.

CDC. 2003a. *An Explanation of U.S. Physical Activity Surveys.* www.cdc.gov/nccdphp/dnpa/physical/physical_surveys.htm. Accessed Dec. 6, 2003.

CDC. 2003b. *Physical Activity and Good Nutrition: Essential Elements to Prevent Chronic Diseases and Obesity.* www.cdc.gov/nccdphp/aag/aag_dnpa.htm. Accessed Nov. 28, 2003.

CDC. 2003c. Physical Activity Levels Among Children Aged 9–13 Years—United States, 2002. *Morbidity and Mortality Weekly Report,* Vol. 52, No. 33, pp. 785–788.

CDC. 2003d. Prevalence of Physical Activity, Including Lifestyle Activities Among Adults—United States, 2000–2001. *Morbidity and Mortality Weekly Report,* Vol. 52, No. 32, pp. 764–769.

DHHS. 1980. *Promoting Health/Preventing Disease: Objectives for the Nation.* Public Health Service, Washington, D.C.

DHHS. 1996. *Physical Activity and Health: A Report of the Surgeon General.* Office of the Surgeon General, Centers for Disease Control and Prevention, Atlanta, Ga.

DHHS. 2000. *Healthy People 2010.* Office of Disease Prevention and Health Promotion, Washington, D.C.

DHHS. 2002. *Physical Activity Fundamental to Preventing Disease.* Office of the Assistant Secretary for Planning and Evaluation, Washington, D.C., June.

Escobedo, L. G., S. E. Marcus, D. Holtzman, and G. A. Giovino. 1993. Sports Participation, Age at Smoking Initiation and the Risk of Smoking Among U.S. High School Students. *Journal of the American Medical Association,* Vol. 269, pp. 1391–1395.

Granner, M. L., and P. A. Sharpe. 2004. Monitoring Physical Activity: Uses and Measurement Issues with Automated Counters. *Journal of Physical Activity and Health,* Vol. 1, pp. 131–141.

Hahn, R. A., S. M. Teutsch, R. B. Rothenberg, and J. S. Marks. 1990. Excess Deaths from Nine Chronic Diseases in the United States, 1986. *Journal of the American Medical Association,* Vol. 264, pp. 2654–2659.

Ham, S. A., M. M. Yore, J. E. Fulton, and H. W. Kohl. 2004. Prevalence of No Leisure-Time Physical Activity—35 States and the District of Columbia, 1988–2002. *Morbidity and Mortality Weekly Report,* Feb. 6, pp. 82–86.

Helmrich, S. P., D. R. Ragland, R. W. Leung, and R. S. Paffenbarger, Jr. 1991. Physical Activity and Reduced Occurrence of Non-Insulin-Dependent Diabetes Mellitus. *New England Journal of Medicine,* Vol. 325, pp. 147–152.

IOM. 2002. *Dietary Reference Intakes for Energy, Carbohydrate, Fiber, Fat, Fatty Acids, Cholesterol, Protein, and Amino Acids.* Prepublication copy, National Academies Press, Washington, D.C.

IOM. 2004. *Preventing Childhood Obesity: Health in the Balance.* National Academies Press, Washington, D.C.

Kaplan, G. A., W. J. Strawbridge, R. D. Cohen, and L. R. Hungerford. 1996. Natural History of Leisure-Time Physical Activity and Its Correlates: Associations with Mortality from All Causes and Cardiovascular Diseases over 28 Years. *American Journal of Epidemiology,* Vol. 144, No. 8, pp. 793–797.

Kraus, W. E., J. A. Houmard, B. D. Duscha, K. J. Knetzger, M. B. Wharton, J. S. McCartney, C. W. Bales, S. Henes, G. P. Samsa, J. D. Otvos, K. R. Kulkarni, and C. A. Slentz. 2002. Effects of the Amount and Intensity of Exercise on Plasma Lipoproteins. *New England Journal of Medicine,* Vol. 347, pp. 1483–1492.

Landers, D. M., and S. M. Arent. 2001. Physical Activity and Mental Health. In *Handbook of Sport Psychology,* 2nd ed. (R. N. Singer, H. A. Hausenblas, and C. M. Janelle, eds.), John Wiley and Sons, New York, pp. 740–765.

Lee, C. D., S. N. Blair, and A. S. Jackson. 1999. Cardiorespiratory Fitness, Body Composition, and All-Cause and Cardiovascular Disease Mortality in Men. *American Journal of Clinical Nutrition,* Vol. 69, pp. 373–380.

Leon, A. S., J. Connett, D. R. Jacobs, Jr., and R. Rauramaa. 1987. Leisure-Time Physical Activity Levels and Risk of Coronary Heart Disease and Death: The Multiple Risk Factor Intervention Trial. *Journal of the American Medical Association,* Vol. 258, pp. 2388–2395.

Manson, J. E., P. Greenland, A. Z. LaCroix, M. L. Stefanick, C. P. Moutton, A. Oberman, M. G. Perri, D. S. Sheps, M. B. Pettinger, and D. S. Siscovick. 2002. Walking Compared with Vigorous Exercise for the Prevention of Cardiovascular Events in Women. *New England Journal of Medicine,* Vol. 347, pp. 716–725.

McGinnis, J. M., and W. H. Foege. 1993. Actual Causes of Death in the United States. *Journal of the American Medical Association,* Vol. 270, No. 18, pp. 2207–2212.

Myers, J., M. Prakahs, V. Froelicher, D. Do, S. Partington, and J. E. Atwood. 2002. Exercise Capacity and Mortality Among Men Referred for Exercise Testing. *New England Journal of Medicine,* Vol. 346, pp. 793–801.

NASPE Council on Physical Education for Children. 2004. *Physical Activity for Children: A Statement of Guidelines for Children Ages 5–12,* 2nd ed.

NCHS. 1989. Design Issues and Alternatives in Assessing Physical Fitness Among Apparently Healthy Adults in a Health Examination Survey of the General Population. In *Assessing Physical Fitness and Physical Activity in Population-Based Surveys,* Department of Health and Human Services, Hyattsville, Md., pp. 107–153.

NCHS. 2003. *Physical Activity Among Adults: United States, 2000.* Advanced Data 333, May 14.

Paffenbarger, R. S., Jr., R. T. Hyde, A. L. Wing, and C.-C. Hsieh. 1986. Physical Activity, All-Cause Mortality, and Longevity of College Alumni. *New England Journal of Medicine,* Vol. 314, pp. 605–613.

Paffenbarger, R. S., Jr., R. T. Hyde, A. L. Wing, I.-M. Lee, D. L. Jung, and J. B. Kampert. 1993. The Association of Changes in Physical-Activity Level and Other Lifestyle Characteristics with Mortality Among Men. *New England Journal of Medicine,* Vol. 328, No. 8, pp. 538–545.

Park, R. J. 1989. *Measurement of Physical Fitness: A Historical Perspective.* Office of Disease Prevention and Health Promotion Monograph Series, Department of Health and Human Services, Washington, D.C., pp. 1–35.

Pate, R. R. 1983. A New Definition of Youth Fitness. *Physician and Sportsmedicine,* Vol. 11, pp. 77–83.

Pate, R. R., G. W. Heath, M. Dowda, and S. G. Trost. 1996. Associations Between Physical Activity and Other Health Behaviors in a Representative Sample of U.S. Adolescents. *American Journal of Public Health,* Vol. 86, No. 11, pp. 1577–1581.

Pate, R. R., M. Pratt, S. N. Blair, W. L. Haskell, C. A. Macera, C. Bouchard, D. Buchner, W. Ettinger, G. W. Heath, A. C. King, A. Kriska, A. S. Leon, B. H. Marcus, J. Morris, R. S. Paffenbarger, Jr., K. Patrick, M. L. Pollock, J. M. Rippe, J. Sallis, and J. H. Wilmore. 1995. Physical Activity and Public Health: A Recommendation from the Centers for Disease Control and Prevention and the American College of Sports Medicine. *Journal of the American Medical Association,* Vol. 273, pp. 402–407.

Powell, K., and S. Blair. 1994. The Public Health Burden of Sedentary Living Habits: Theoretical but Realistic Estimates. *Medicine and Science in Sports and Exercise,* Vol. 26, No. 7, pp. 851–856.

Report to the President. 2000. *Promoting Better Health for Young People Through Physical Activity and Sports: A Report to the President from the Secretary of Health and Human Services and the Secretary of Education.* Department of Health and Human Services, Department of Education, Silver Spring, Md.

Sallis, J. F., T. L. McKenzie, B. Kolody, M. Lewis, S. Marshall, and P. Rosengard. 1999. Effects of Health-Related Physical Education on Academic Performance: Project SPARK. *Research Quarterly for Exercise and Sport,* Vol. 70, No. 2, pp. 127–134.

Sherman, S. E., R. B. D'Agostino, J. L. Cobb, and W. B. Kannel. 1994. Physical Activity and Mortality in Women in the Framingham Heart Study. *American Heart Journal,* Vol. 128, No. 5, pp. 879–884.

Slattery, M. L., D. R. Jacobs, Jr., and N. Z. Nichaman. 1989. Leisure-Time Physical Activity and Coronary Heart Disease Death: The U.S. Railroad Study. *Circulation,* Vol. 79, pp. 304–311.

Vainio, H., and F. Bianchini (eds.). 2002. Weight Control and Physical Activity. *IARC Handbooks of Cancer Prevention,* IARC Press, Vol. 6.

Wei, M., J. B. Kampert, C. E. Barlow, M. Z. Nichaman, L. W. Gibbons, R. S. Paffenbarger, Jr., and S. N. Blair. 1999. Relationship Between Low Cardiorespiratory Fitness and Mortality in Normal-Weight, Overweight, and Obese Men. *Journal of the American Medical Association,* Vol. 282, pp. 1547–1553.

WHO. 1946. Preamble to the Constitution of the World Health Organization as adopted by the International Health Conference, New York, June 19–22. *Official Records of the World Health Organization,* Vol. 2, p. 100.

Wilson, P. W. F., R. S. Paffenbarger, J. N. Morris, and R. J. Havlik. 1986. Assessment Methods of Physical Activity and Physical Fitness in Population Studies: A Report of an NHLBI Workshop. *American Heart Journal,* Vol. 111, pp. 1177–1192.

Zill, N., C. W. Nord, and L. S. Loomis. 1995. *Adolescent Time Use, Risky Behavior and Outcomes: An Analysis of National Data.* Westat, Rockville, Md.

SUMMARY

Long-Term Trends Affecting Physical Activity Levels

T he trend data reviewed in this chapter show that technological innovations, as well as broad social and economic changes, have steadily and substantially reduced the physical demands of work, home, and travel, with a modest and recent offset in increased leisure-time, higher-intensity physical activity for some sectors of the population. Long-term changes in the built environment have also contributed to declining physical activity levels. The suburbanization of the population and employment in lower-density communities and office locations have increased reliance on private vehicles for most trips.

Available trend data, particularly on the role of the built environment in declining levels of physical activity, are limited in their explanatory power. First, the indicators are too general to illuminate how land use patterns and travel affect an individual's decision to be physically active. Second, some of the key data of interest, for example, information on nonmotorized travel, are available but have not been collected with any reliability until very recently. Where trend data are directly available, more analysis is needed to determine whether observed changes are indeed significantly different in a statistical sense. Finally, with the possible exception of time-use data, available trend data do not provide an integrated perspective on the environmental factors affecting physical activity levels or on the trade-offs among them. For example, walking has declined as a mode of transport to work but may be on the increase for recreational purposes. The net effect on total physical activity levels, however, is unclear. In sum, the longitudinal data are suggestive but not definitive regarding the many factors contributing to changes in total physical activity levels.

Time-use data may best help frame the opportunities and limitations of various strategies for increasing total physical activity to meet the 30-minute daily minimum. For example, doubling the use of nonmotorized transportation would increase daily physical activity levels associated with travel to an average of only 6 minutes at the population level. Work provides another potential opportunity for increasing physical activity, for example, through short exercise breaks and lunchtime walks. Finally, more active use of free time—reducing the time spent watching television and engaging in other sedentary activities or augmenting the time already spent by those who participate in sports and exercise—offers another important opportunity for increasing daily physical activity levels. For many, a combination of small increments in physical activity in many locations may be the most feasible way of meeting the daily requirement.

3

Long-Term Trends Affecting Physical Activity Levels

The previous chapter revealed that the majority of the U.S. population is not meeting recommended guidelines for physical activity and that a sizeable fraction characterizes itself as completely inactive or sedentary. This chapter takes a longer view to determine whether there is evidence of a growing problem, and, as the available data permit, traces trends in technology introduction and other social and economic changes over the past 50 years or longer that may help explain current inadequate levels of physical activity.

ANALYSIS APPROACH

An ideal starting point in attempting to sort out the complex links between physical activity and the built environment would be to examine long-term trends and data related to physical activity, travel behavior, and urban form. Researchers are immediately confronted, however, with the lack of direct measures and longitudinal data even on changes in physical activity levels—the primary variable of interest. Until 2001, for example, major public health surveys tracked data on leisure-time physical activity only, and reliable data were not collected until the 1980s. Trend data on physical activity at home, at work, and in transport are unavailable (see Figure 1-2 in Chapter 1, which defines the four types of physical activity of interest). Thus, it is not possible to track directly how total physical activity levels have changed over time.

Faced with this challenge, the committee commissioned a paper (Brownson and Boehmer 2004) to examine historical trends and societal changes affecting physical activity from which meaningful associations and shifts in behavior could be inferred over time. For example, quantitative trend data are not available on physical activity in the workplace. However, labor force data that enable occupations to be classified by activity level can be used to trace occupational changes from 1950 to 2000. From these data, one can draw inferences, at least at a gross level, about changes in physical activity levels in the workplace.

Another line of inquiry is to examine time use. Time is a scarce and constrained commodity (i.e., a day has 24 hours regardless of other changes). How individuals allocate their time among a range of activities provides useful insights about their opportunities for and propensity to engage in physical activity. Data on time use are available from analyses of detailed diaries dating back to 1965 and conducted every decade since (Robinson and Godbey 1999).[1] These analyses enable direct observation of changes in physical activity levels over time, such as time spent on recreational activities (e.g., active sports, walking, cycling, other fitness activities). The analyses also document changes in time use and time availability with more indirect implications for physical activity. For example, time spent on housework has declined steadily since 1965—the result of technological improvements in the home (e.g., availability of prepared foods) and increased participation of women in the workforce (Cutler et al. 2003). These data suggest a loss in physical activity for some women due to a reduction in household chores, such as housecleaning. However, the change has also freed up time that, in theory, could be used for exercise or the pursuit of other leisure-time physical activities.

---

[1] The 1965 and 1975 surveys were conducted by the Institute for Social Research at the University of Michigan, and the 1985 and 1995 surveys by the Survey Research Center at the University of Maryland. The key methodological features of the time diary analyses are summarized by Robinson and Godbey (1999, Table 32).

TRENDS IN LEISURE-TIME PHYSICAL ACTIVITY

Reliable trend data on leisure-time physical activity levels for U.S. adults and adolescents have been collected since 1990.[2] Data from the Behavioral Risk Factor Surveillance Survey (BRFSS) show a slight gain in meeting recommended levels of physical activity and a complementary decline in reported physical inactivity for U.S. adults from 1990 to 2000 (see Figure 3-1). In 1990, approximately 24 percent of adults met recommended physical activity levels and in 2000, about 26 percent—a compound average annual growth rate of 0.75 percent. For the same period, nearly 31 percent of adults reported they were inactive in 1990; that is, they did not engage in any leisure-time physical activity. By 2000, that figure had fallen to nearly 28 percent—a compound average annual rate of decline of 1.06 percent.

The BRFSS data show improvements in physical activity levels for both men and women from 1990 to 2000 (Brownson and Boehmer 2004). However, analysis of the data by educational level and race reveals diverging trends. For example, those with less than 12 years of education showed a small but persistent decline in meeting recommended physical activity guidelines compared with those with a college education or at least some college. Non-Hispanic whites and blacks showed modest gains in meeting the guidelines, but Hispanic adults registered a slight decline.[3]

Trend data from the National Health Interview Survey (NHIS) for the period 1985 to 1998 show results similar to those of the BRFSS, that is, a slight improvement in the percentage of adults meeting recommended levels of physical activity. However, the NHIS data show essentially stable rates of inactive behavior (see Figure 3-2).

---

[2] This section draws heavily on the paper by Brownson and Boehmer (2004) commissioned for this study. Although earlier data are available from the BRFSS, only even-year data for 1990–2000 were used because the surveys in these years sampled at least 43 states and the District of Columbia and are considered to be the most reliable (Brownson and Boehmer 2004). More recent data from the 2001 survey were not used because of the changes made in the questionnaire to obtain a more complete picture of physical activity levels (see Chapter 2).

[3] These data are shown graphically in Figures 2 through 4 of the Brownson and Boehmer paper.

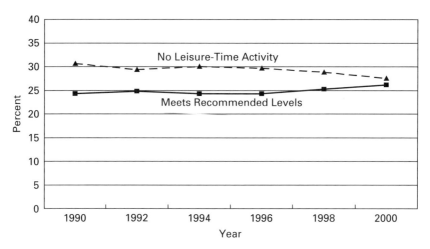

FIGURE 3-1 **Percentage of U.S. adult population meeting recommended physical activity levels or reported as inactive.**
(SOURCE: BRFSS 1990–2000.)

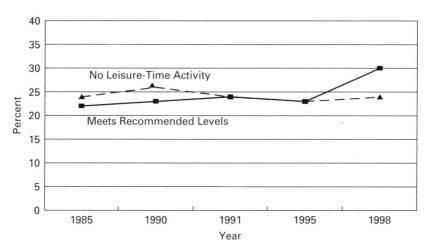

FIGURE 3-2 **Percentage of U.S. adult population meeting recommended physical activity levels or reporting no leisure-time physical activity.**
(SOURCE: NHIS 1985–1998.)

As noted, time-use diaries provide a longer-term perspective on changes in leisure-time activities. In 1995, survey respondents reported spending nearly 50 minutes a day in active sports, outdoor activities, walking, cycling, and other exercise for recreation—an increase of about 20 minutes a day since the 1965 survey (Cutler et al. 2003).

Trend data on physical activity levels among youth are also available. The Youth Risk Behavior Survey System (YRBSS) data for 1991–2001 show that rates of vigorous activity for high school students (i.e., vigorous physical activity for 20 minutes or more at least three times a week) remained constant over the decade of the 1990s (see Figure 3-3). The percentage of students attending physical education classes daily—an indicator of physical activity levels—declined sharply during the first half of the decade, but increased gradually thereafter (Figure 3-3).

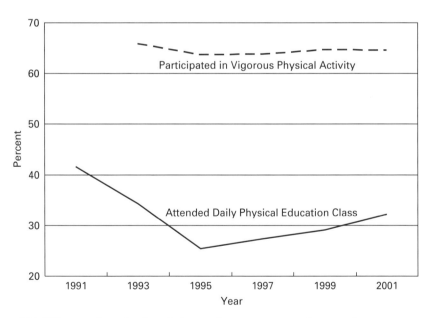

FIGURE 3-3   **Physical activity indicators in youths, grades 9 through 12.**
(Source: YRBSS 1991–2001.)

No systematic trend data are available on changes in children's physical activity levels. However, there has been a decline in walking and cycling to school (EPA 2003), and there is some evidence that children spend less time in play outdoors (IOM 2004).

In sum, these data show that U.S. adults made modest gains in the pursuit of leisure-time physical activity over the past decade, while physical activity levels among youths appear to have remained unchanged. To obtain a more complete picture of changes in total physical activity levels, however, it is necessary to examine broader structural changes in the economy and society.

TRENDS IN OTHER TYPES OF PHYSICAL ACTIVITY

The twentieth century can be characterized as the century of technological change (Brownson and Boehmer 2004). The growth of white-collar jobs in the workplace, the introduction of labor-saving devices in the home, and the widespread use of the automobile as the primary form of transport have resulted in a pervasive reduction in the physical demands of daily life. Table 3-1 provides a time line of many technological innovations and supporting systems linked to reduced daily energy expenditure and increased opportunities for leisure-time sedentary activities (e.g., watching television, using the computer). The time line covers a longer period than most of the other trend data presented in this chapter, which are focused on the latter half of the twentieth century.

Employment and Occupational Changes

Between 1950 and 2000, the surge of women into the workforce, the continued decline in agricultural employment and manufacturing jobs, and other technological and social changes conducive to the growth of white-collar jobs brought about profound changes in physical activity levels in the workplace. The U.S. civilian labor force more than doubled from about 62 million in 1950 to about 143 million in 2000 (Brownson and Boehmer 2004). Participation by women increased by a factor of 3.6 compared with a factor of 1.7

TABLE 3-1 Twentieth-Century Technological Innovations and Supporting Systems

Time Interval	Work	Home Production/Food	Transport and Land Use	Communications
1900–1925		1901: vacuum cleaner invented 1923: frozen food invented circa 1925: first electric washer, automatic washer, and automatic dryer	1900: modern escalator invented 1903: Wright Brothers invent the first engined airplane 1904: invention of the tractor 1906: first Mack trucks built 1908: Henry Ford improves the assembly line, and the first Model T is sold 1916: first Federal-Aid Road Act 1923: traffic signal invented	1916: first radio tuners that receive different stations invented 1923: television cathode-ray tube invented
1926–1950		1946: microwave oven invented 1949: cake mix invented	1930: jet engine invented 1940: first freeway in California from Pasadena to Los Angeles 1949: Levittown	1927: first successful talking motion picture 1939: first scheduled television broadcasts 1949: network television starts in the United States
1951–1975	1950: first automatic elevators 1958: photocopier invented 1962: introduction of first industrial robot 1972: word processor invented	1954: first McDonald's; first TV dinner introduced 1964: permanent press fabric invented 1971: food processor invented	1952: first jet airliner for commercial passenger service 1956: Federal-Aid Highway Act and beginning of the Interstate highway system 1963: first people mover introduced in the United States	1951: computers first sold commercially 1955: first wireless TV remote invented 1958: integrated circuit invented 1959: microchip invented 1968: first computer with integrated circuits 1971: microprocessor invented; videocassette recorder invented
1976–2000				1976: Apple home computer invented 1981: first IBM PC sold 1990: World Wide Web/Internet protocol and language created

SOURCES: Twentieth-Century Inventions 1900–1999, History of Transportation, History of Communication (inventors.about.com, accessed June 6, 2004); Bruno 1993.

for men, presumably with a large increase in lower-activity, white-collar jobs. Agricultural employment, typically a high-activity occupation, continued to decline from 12 percent of the labor force in 1950 to 2 percent in 2000. In nonagricultural establishments, the number of employees engaged in manufacturing fell sharply from 30 to 13 percent between 1950 and 2000, while those in the service sector—with a higher fraction of less physically demanding white-collar jobs—grew from about two-fifths to nearly four-fifths of civilian employment over the same period (BLS 2004a).

Occupational data from the U.S. census categorized by activity level for this same time period show the results of these major structural changes.[4] The share of the eligible labor force in low-activity occupations nearly doubled from 1950 to 2000, with the majority of that shift taking place in the first 20 years (see Figure 3-4). Today, approximately one-quarter of the eligible labor force, or 58.2 million people, is employed in low-activity occupations (Brownson and Boehmer 2004). The proportion of high-activity occupations remained relatively stable at 16 to 17 percent of the eligible labor force over this period, but then declined to about 14 percent from 1990 to 2000 (Figure 3-4). Today, about 31 million people are employed in high-activity occupations.

It is not possible to characterize the occupations of the remaining 59 percent of the eligible labor force or to disaggregate the data by gender or other demographic variables. Nevertheless, the available data show major shifts in the tails of the distribution, which suggest a generally downward trend in physical activity levels in the workplace. In 1950, approximately 30 percent more of the labor force was engaged in high-activity than in low-activity occupations. By 2000, roughly twice as many persons were employed in low-activity than in high-activity occupations (Brownson and Boehmer 2004).

---

[4] Brownson and Boehmer took occupational data from the U.S. census that had been recoded by researchers at the University of Minnesota Population Center to enhance compatibility in job classifications across years, and categorized the data by activity level on the basis of occupational descriptions contained in the 1988–1994 National Health and Nutrition Examination Survey III database. For more detail, see Brownson and Boehmer 2004.

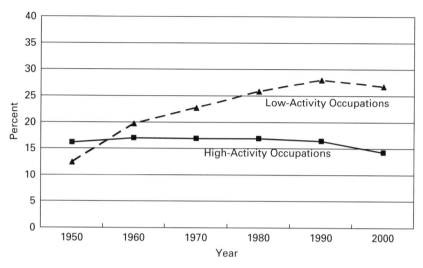

FIGURE 3-4 **Occupations classified by activity level, percent of eligible labor force at least 16 years old, 1950–2000.** (Source: Brownson and Boehmer 2004, Figure 8.)

Changes in Household Activities

The sharp increase in women in the labor force, along with the introduction of labor-saving technology improvements in the home, has resulted in major changes in the time and energy devoted to household production. These changes in turn have important implications for physical activity levels. Foremost among these changes is the decline in time spent on housework and other moderate-level activities in the home. Longitudinal data from time diaries show that for women, time spent on household activities, including housework (e.g., housecleaning, laundry, meal preparation and cleanup), shopping, and child care, fell by nearly one-third from 1965 to 1995, from about 40 to about 27 hours per week (Robinson and Godbey 1999). Although the trend for men is in the opposite direction, overall the data indicate a net reduction in time devoted to household and family care, with the decline in housework being the dominant explanatory factor (Robinson and Godbey 1999). Thus, physical activity associated with housework is on the decline, at least for women. What is less clear is how women, and to a lesser extent men, are using the time thus made available, a topic discussed in a subsequent section. Other changes in household structure (e.g., increasing numbers of single-person households, activity patterns and sharing of dual-worker households) are also likely to affect the time allocated to physical activity.

Changes in Travel Behavior

Personal transport in the twentieth century has been dominated by the introduction and growth of automobile travel. In 2001, respondents to the household interview for the National Household Travel Survey (NHTS) reported that, for the first time, the number of personal vehicles per household (1.9) exceeded the mean number of reported drivers per household (1.8) (BTS 2003). In 1969, there were 1.2 reported personal vehicles per household and 1.6 reported licensed drivers per household (Hu and Young 1999). According to the U.S. census, the proportion of households owning more than one vehicle in 2000 was more than double that reported in 1960, a reflection of both the increased disposable personal income and the preferences of the U.S. population (Brownson and Boehmer 2004).

Not surprisingly, increased vehicle ownership and improvements in highway infrastructure, among other factors, have been associated with a sharp increase in personal travel, although the dominant direction of causality is not clear. The 2001 NHTS reported about 4 trillion person miles of travel, an average of about 14, 500 miles per person annually (BTS 2003). In 1969, 1.4 trillion person miles of travel was reported, for an annual per person average of about 7,100 (DOT 2001).

The vast majority of trips are made by passenger vehicle, and this has been true for decades. In 1995, respondents to the Nationwide Personal Transportation Survey (NPTS)—the precursor to the current NHTS—reported making approximately 87 percent of daily trips for all purposes in a personal vehicle; in 1977, the equiv-

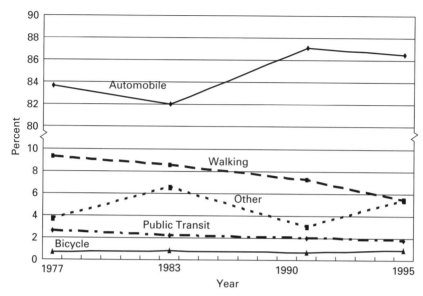

FIGURE 3-5 **Percentage of trips by transport mode for U.S. daily travel, all trip purposes, 1977–1995. "Other" includes primarily school bus trips, as well as trips by taxicab, ferry, airplane, and helicopter.**
(SOURCE: Pucher and Renne 2003, 51.)

alent number was 84 percent (Pucher and Renne 2003) (see Figure 3-5).[5] The journey-to-work data from the U.S. census, which provide comparable data for a longer period, show increasing reliance on the automobile for commutes. In 1960, roughly two-thirds of such trips were made by car; by 2000, this share had grown to more than four-fifths (Pucher and Renne 2003) (see Figure 3-6). For all trips, the average amount of time spent daily in driving reported by all drivers has increased steadily in recent years—in part because of increased travel and in part because of greater road congestion. Comparable data for 1990–2001 alone show a growth in

---

[5] Data from the 1969 survey were not included because walking and bicycle trips were not sampled, so the shares of motorized travel were artificially inflated. Data from the 2001 survey were not included because of a change in sampling methods that captures previously unreported walking trips (Pucher and Renne 2003).

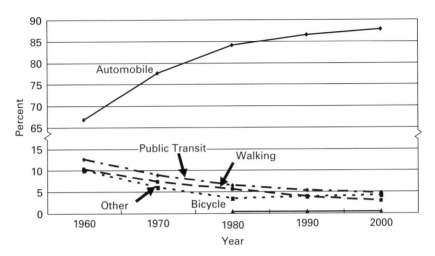

FIGURE 3-6   **Percentage of trips by transport mode for U.S. work trips, 1960–2000. "Other" includes "work at home" and "all other."**
(SOURCE: Pucher and Renne 2003, 50.)

the average time spent driving from 49 to 62 minutes per day (Hu and Young 1999).[6]

Corresponding to the growth in personal vehicle travel, non-motorized travel—primarily walking and cycling but also trips on public transportation that require some walking or cycling to access rail stations and bus stops—has declined over time (Figures 3-5 and 3-6). Gathering reliable data on nonmotorized travel, particularly walking and cycling, however, has not been a priority in U.S. travel surveys, and thus these modes of travel have not been well measured. When a concerted effort was made in the 2001 NHTS to obtain a more complete accounting of walking trips, the share of such trips increased to nearly 9 percent—second only to automobile trips (BTS 2003). The percentage of walking trips was found to be in-

---

[6] Data from the NHTS for 2001 were accessed online by using the Oak Ridge National Laboratory website (nhts.ornl.gov/2001). The figures reported here represent the average time spent driving a private vehicle reported by all drivers. They exclude driving in segmented trips or as an essential part of work (Hu and Young 1999). Segmented trips are defined as trips that involve a change of vehicle or mode, with one of the modes used involving public transportation (e.g., bus, subway).

TABLE 3-2   Percentage of Urban Trips by Transportation Mode and Trip Purpose, Calculated from the 2001 National Household Travel Survey

Transportation Mode	Trip Purpose			
	Work and Work-Related	Shopping and Services	Social and Recreation	School and Church
Automobile	92.1	91.5	84.1	72.9
Transit	3.7	1.4	1.0	2.2
Walking	3.4	6.5	12.7	10.5
Bicycle	0.5	0.3	1.3	0.7
Other	0.3	0.3	0.8	13.8

NOTE: "Other" includes school bus, taxicab, and all other.
SOURCE: Pucher and Renne 2003, 53.

versely related to automobile ownership, income level, and being of a minority race (often correlated with income). Walking represented a greater share of trips for those who reported not owning a car, for those in the lowest income bracket (≤$20,000), and for nonwhite respondents (Pucher and Renne 2003).

The importance of nonmotorized travel also varied by trip purpose. The 2001 NHTS found the highest levels of walking and cycling on trips for social and recreational purposes and to school and church. Public transit was used most for work and work-related trips (Pucher and Renne 2003) (see Table 3-2). At the same time, the automobile continues to be the dominant form of transport for all trip types.[7]

Travel surveys also show a sharp decline in walking and cycling to school. In 1969, the NPTS reported that 48 percent of students walked or cycled to school (EPA 2003). The 2001 NHTS found that less than 15 percent of students between the ages of 5 and 15 walked to or from school, and only 1 percent cycled (EPA 2003).[8] As discussed in Chapter 2, the NHTS results are higher for those who live

---

[7] Analysis of the 2001 NHTS revealed that only 8 percent of households reported not having a car. The vast majority of these reported a household income of <$20,000 (Pucher and Renne 2003).

[8] The Environmental Protection Agency reports that the 1969 figure applies to students in elementary and intermediate grades, the closest counterparts to the 5–15 age range reported in 2001 (EPA 2003).

within 1 to 2 miles of school. Nevertheless, the vast majority of children travel to and from school in automobiles, vans, and school or transit buses (TRB 2002).

Summary of Effects on Physical Activity Levels

The trend data reviewed in this section, although indirect, point to a substantial decline in physical activity levels in the workplace, at home, and in travel over a long period. The following sections examine other factors that may help explain this decline, including trends in the spatial distributions of population and employment and in time use, particularly the growth in sedentary activities.

TRENDS IN SPATIAL DISTRIBUTIONS OF POPULATION AND EMPLOYMENT

In examining the built environment as a possible explanation for at least some of the observed decline in physical activity levels, the focus is often on the effect of low-density development on the proximity of travel destinations, which in turn influences transportation choices.

Two major trends characterized the spatial distribution of population throughout the past century. The first is the population shift from rural to metropolitan areas, or metropolitan statistical areas (MSAs) as they are termed by the U.S. Bureau of the Census.[9] In 1900, the U.S. population was predominately rural; by 2000, 80 percent of the population lived in metropolitan areas (see Figure 3-7). The second trend is the movement within metropolitan areas from central cities to the suburbs. Suburbanization trends can be traced back at least to the 1880s, with increases in suburban population growth following World War I and World War II (NRC 1999). In

---

[9] MSAs are statistical geographic entities consisting of at least one core urbanized area with a population of at least 50,000. The MSA comprises the central county or counties containing the core, plus adjacent outlying counties with a high degree of social and economic integration with the central county, as measured by commuting ties with the counties containing the core (*Federal Register* 2000). Of course, boundaries of MSAs change over time. Decennial census data reflect MSA boundaries defined at the time of each census year.

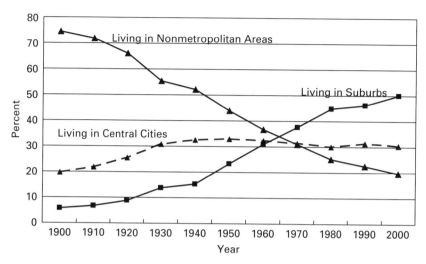

FIGURE 3-7   **Percentage of total population living in central cities and suburbs of metropolitan areas and in nonmetropolitan areas, 1900–2000.**
(SOURCE: Decennial Census of Population, U.S. Bureau of the Census.)

1950, for example, slightly more than one-fifth of the population lived in suburbs. By 2000, this number had more than doubled, largely at the expense of nonmetropolitan areas; central cities have maintained their current share of the population—approximately 30 percent—over a long period of time (NRC 1999) (Figure 3-7). The long-term suburbanization of the U.S. population can be traced to broad economic, social, and political changes, as well as the role of federal mortgage insurance programs of the 1950s, the expansion of the Interstate highway system in the 1960s, and the fiscal and social problems of the cities in the 1960s and 1970s (NRC 1999).[10]

---

[10] The economic and social changes encompass technological changes that enabled employment to decentralize, increases in household income that allowed households to act on their preferences for greater space, and improvements in transportation infrastructure that reduced commuting costs. Political changes include the political separation of city and suburbs, which resulted from the opposition of middle-class neighborhoods at the city's edge to expanding the city boundaries in order to annex these communities and passage of state laws permitting easy municipal incorporation (NRC 1999).

Jobs have followed population to the suburbs. In 1950, about 70 percent of jobs were located in central cities; by 1990, that figure had fallen to 45 percent (Mieszkowski and Mills 1993). Furthermore, since World War II, employment—and, to a lesser extent, population—has grown more rapidly in small and less dense MSAs.[11] This trend is referred to as deconcentration and has been attributed primarily to the costs of congestion—both higher living costs for households and higher production costs for firms (Carlino 2000). The result has been a more uniform spatial distribution of employment and population both within and across MSAs, although the largest and densest MSAs still account for the highest share of total population and employment (Carlino 2000).

Metropolitan areas can also be characterized by spatial clustering in central cities with respect to both race and income (Berube and Tiffany 2004; NRC 1999). Minority and poor populations live disproportionately in central cities rather than in suburbs, a situation reflecting racial as well as economic segregation (NRC 1999).[12] The concentration of the poor in the ghettos and barrios of central cities magnifies the social ills that accompany poverty and has exacerbated the flight of middle- and higher-income populations to the suburbs, further magnifying the concentration effect (Jargowsky 2003). High-poverty neighborhoods typically exhibit a cycle of disinvestment and decay—gradually declining investments in housing, commerce, and infrastructure; reductions in public services (e.g., garbage pickup, bus service); loss of established institutions (e.g., banks and supermarkets); and loss of population. Between 1970 and 1990, both the number and share of people living in high-poverty neighborhoods (i.e., neighborhoods where the poverty rate is 40 percent or higher) rose sharply in many MSAs. With the exception of the Hispanic population, however, the incidence of those living in high-poverty neighborhoods declined by nearly

---

[11] Density is measured as employment or population per square mile.

[12] The residential racial segregation of blacks is not simply a by-product of economic segregation. Massey and Denton (1993) found that high-income blacks live in areas nearly as segregated as those populated by low-income blacks, while the segregation of Hispanics and Asians falls steadily as income rises.

one-quarter during the 1990s, as did the concentration of poverty. Blacks and Native Americans showed the largest declines on both measures in central cities and rural areas, respectively. Nevertheless, in 2000, blacks remained the single largest group living in high-poverty neighborhoods, and both blacks and Native Americans exhibited the highest concentrated poverty rates (Jargowsky 2003).

Spatial concentration by income and race has been a constant feature of the built environment, but the location of these groups has shifted over time. After World War II, policies of urban renewal, central city revitalization, and gentrification resulted in the displacement of poor populations mainly within central cities, but often from the central core. This process of dispersion has continued, most recently with the movement of many minority groups to the older suburbs (U.S. Bureau of the Census 2002). In fact, the inner-ring suburbs were the only geographic areas that did not show a decline in the number of high-poverty neighborhoods between 1990 and 2000, and many experienced increases in poverty over the decade (Jargowsky 2003).

What do these trends imply for travel, particularly by nonmotorized modes? First, geographic characterization of the spatial dimensions of the built environment according to central cities, suburbs, and nonmetropolitan areas falls short of capturing the complexity of urban settings (e.g., ghetto neighborhoods in inner cities, inner suburbs, "edge cities,"[13] exurban areas) and the ways in which these differences may affect residents' propensity to be physically active. For example, the concentration of development in edge cities may be sufficiently compact to support public transit and encourage walking and cycling to some destinations. In contrast, large residential suburban developments without sidewalks or bicycle trails and with cul-de-sac street layouts may make driving the only reasonable alternative for most trips.

Second, suburbanization of the population should decrease the accessibility, that is, the proximity and convenience, of many

---

[13] The term "edge cities," coined by *Washington Post* journalist and author Joel Garreau in 1991, refers to suburban cities, typically located near major freeway intersections.

destinations, thereby increasing the reliance on more time-saving automobile travel for many trip purposes. Data from the 2001 American Housing Survey suggest that a sizeable fraction of the U.S. population still lives in settings with destinations that could be reached by nonmotorized modes. For example, nearly two-thirds of survey respondents reported having satisfactory neighborhood shopping within 1 mile of their home. Fifty-five percent reported having access to public transit, and among U.S. residents with children ≤13 years old, nearly 57 percent had a public elementary school within 1 mile of their residence. However, when the data are analyzed by geographic characteristics—central cities and suburban areas within MSAs and areas outside of MSAs—more densely populated central cities exhibit higher levels of access, which offer their residents greater opportunities for non-motorized travel (see Table 3-3). Unfortunately, these data are available only for the 1997, 1999, and 2001 surveys, which makes any meaningful trend analysis impossible. Furthermore, the level of detail is insufficient to indicate the characteristics of particular locations that might encourage walking or cycling or taking transit to accessible destinations.

TABLE 3-3   Selected Access Measures for Neighborhood-Occupied Housing Units by Geographic Area

	In MSAs (%)		
Selected Access Measure	**Central Cities**	**Suburbs**	**Outside MSAs (%)**
Housing units with public elementary school <1 mile[a]	72	54	40
Housing units with public transportation[b]	82	52	23
Housing units with shopping <1 mile[b]	77	62	41

NOTE: MSA = metropolitan statistical area.
[a] This measure is based on the number of households with children aged 0 to 13—9.2 million in central cities, 16.6 million in suburbs, and 5.6 million outside MSAs.
[b] This measure is based on the total number of occupied housing units—31.7 million in central cities, 53.6 million in suburbs, and 20.9 million outside MSAs.
SOURCE: American Housing Survey, 2001: Neighborhood-Occupied Units, Table 2-8, pp. 58–63.

Finally, the geographic concentration of the poor in central cities generates a host of social ills that accompany poverty—drug trafficking, violent crime, economic (poor access to suburban jobs) and social isolation, limited provision of public services, and poorly maintained infrastructure—that are likely to discourage poor populations from engaging in physical activity except for necessary trips. The effect on physical activity levels of the recent move of poor and minority populations to the inner suburbs is likely to be mixed. The inner suburbs of older cities are apt to look much like their downtowns, with sidewalks and transit service. This may not be true, however, in newer cities, where the inner suburbs may offer less in the way of transit services and physical facilities (e.g., sidewalks). In both cases, crime and public safety are likely to be salient concerns.

CHANGES IN TIME USE AND SEDENTARY ACTIVITIES

A comparison of time use in 1995 and 1965 that combines the results for women and men (Cutler et al. 2003) reveals some gains in free time due to a decline in housework (discussed previously) and, to a lesser extent, declines in eating and personal care time, which could be used in more physically active endeavors (see Figure 3-8). Part of the freed-up time was in fact used for increased recreation—active sports, outdoor activities, walking, hiking, and other exercise. The majority, however, was spent on more television watching and additional hours of sleep (Figure 3-8).[14] Sleeping continues to claim the largest share of available daily time—about one-third on average. Television watching accounts for about another 10 percent of available daily time and has grown to be the dominant leisure-time activity.

A recent analysis of one of the time-use diary surveys from the 1990s used the data on activity type to estimate daily energy

---

[14] Additional daily hours spent sleeping, however, peaked in 1975 and have remained relatively constant over the next two decades.

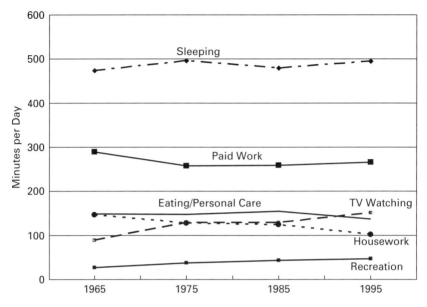

FIGURE 3-8   Time use, 1965–1995 (ages 18–64).
(SOURCE: Cutler et al. 2003.)

expenditure.[15] The results show a picture of daily life in which sedentary and low-intensity activities predominate (Dong et al. 2004). Excluding sleeping, which accounts for nearly one-fifth of the overall energy expenditure of the population, the activities that account for 50 percent of waking-hour energy expenditure, in order of priority, are driving a car, office work, watching television or a movie, taking care of children, sitting, eating, and cleaning house (see Table 3-4). With the exception of taking care of children and cleaning house, these activities are of very light intensity.

---

[15] Data from the National Human Activity Pattern Survey conducted in 1992–1994 were used to estimate and rank the energy expenditure for each activity. Survey respondents reported activities in their own words for a 24-hour period, including the location and duration of the activity. Activities were recoded into 255 categories, which were then assigned appropriate metabolic expenditure values using the Ainsworth compendium and update, respectively (Ainsworth et al. 1993; Ainsworth et al. 2000). A score was created for each activity by multiplying the duration and intensity for each individual and summing across individuals, and then each score was ranked by its contribution to total population energy expenditure. More detail on the calculation of energy expenditure is given by Dong et al. (2004).

TABLE 3-4   Ranking of Activities That Account for 50 Percent of Daily Energy Expenditure in the United States

Rank	Activity Description	MET	Percent of Total Score	Cumulative Percentage
(1)	Sleeping, napping	0.9	(19.1)	—
1	Driving car	2.3	10.9	10.9
2	Job: office work, typing	1.5	9.2	20.1
3	Watching TV/movie, home or theater	1.0	8.6	28.7
4	Taking care of child (feeding, bathing, dressing)	3.0	8.4	37.1
5	Activities performed while sitting quietly	1.3	5.8	42.9
6	Eating (sitting)	1.5	5.3	48.2
7	Cleaning house, general	3.0	3.9	52.1

NOTE: MET = metabolic equivalent (see Chapter 2 for a definition).
SOURCE: Dong et al. 2004.

Leisure-time, high-intensity activities account for less than 3 percent of total waking energy expenditure in this sample population.

In August 2004, the Bureau of Labor Statistics released the results of the first American Time-Use Survey (ATUS). A monthly survey conducted by the U.S. Bureau of the Census, the ATUS will provide a consistent and continuous source of nationally representative daily time-use data that can readily be combined with demographic and employment data, as well as data on energy expenditure.[16] On an "average day" in 2003, persons in the United States aged 15 and older reported that they slept about 8.6 hours, engaged in leisure and sports activities for 5.1 hours, worked for 3.7 hours, and spent 1.8 hours doing household activities.[17] The remaining 4.8 hours was

---

[16] The ATUS was administered to an outrotated panel of the Current Population Survey, thereby providing demographic and labor force information. Data collection began in January 2003, and the ATUS estimates for that year are based on interviews of about 21,000 individuals. The survey was administered to one member of a household (15 years or older), who provided information on activities lasting 5 minutes or longer in the preceding 24-hour period (BLS 2004b).

[17] An average day encompasses both weekdays and weekends and is computed on the basis of all responses from a given population, including respondents who did not engage in a particular activity on their diary day. The activities cited are primary activities, that is, those identified by respondents as their main activity (BLS 2004b).

spent on such activities as eating and drinking, attending school, and shopping (BLS 2004b). These results confirm the findings of the earlier 1995 time-use survey regarding sedentary use of free time. According to the ATUS, the population at large, on average, has approximately 5 free hours available on an average day and spends approximately half of this time watching television. Only 18 minutes on average is spent on sports, exercise, and recreation (BLS 2004b).

Time spent on transportation is not identified separately in the ATUS but is included with the appropriate activity. To estimate time spent on travel, particularly on active travel, that is, on walking, cycling, and accessing public transit, a detailed analysis of the 1995 NPTS was conducted by one of the committee members. The results show that, on average, adults (persons 18 years and older) spend 64 minutes per day traveling by all modes of transport. Of that time, an average of 3 minutes is spent on active travel. The committee recognizes that these results are likely to undercount active travel—detailed analysis of the 2001 NHTS and future surveys should provide better estimates of nonmotorized travel. Nevertheless, the results suggest that active travel represents a small fraction of the total time spent in transportation.

REFERENCES

Abbreviations

BLS	Bureau of Labor Statistics
BTS	Bureau of Transportation Statistics
DOT	U.S. Department of Transportation
EPA	U.S. Environmental Protection Agency
IOM	Institute of Medicine
NRC	National Research Council
TRB	Transportation Research Board

Ainsworth, B. E., W. L. Haskell, A. S. Leon, D. R. Jacobs, Jr., H. J. Montoye, J. F. Sallis, and R. S. Paffenbarger, Jr. 1993. Compendium of Physical Activities: Classification of Energy Costs of Human Physical Activities. *Medicine and Science in Sports and Exercise,* Vol. 25, pp. 71–80.

Ainsworth, B. E., W. L. Haskell, M. C. Whitt, M. L. Irwin, A. M. Swartz, S. J. Strath, W. L. O'Brien, D. R. Bassett, Jr., K. H. Schmitz, P. O. Emplaincourt, D. R. Jacobs, Jr., and A. S. Leon. 2000. Compendium of Physical Activities: An Update of Activity Codes and MET Intensities. *Medicine and Science in Sports and Exercise,* Vol. 32, pp. S498–S504.

Berube, A., and T. Tiffany. 2004. *The Shape of the Curve: Household Income Distributions in U.S. Cities, 1979–1999.* Living Census Series, Metropolitan Policy Program, Brookings Institution, Aug.

BLS. 2004a. *Employment and Earnings.* Table B-1: Employees on Non-Farm Payrolls by Industry Sector and Selected Industry Detail. data.bls.gov/servlet/SurveyOutput Servlet. Accessed March 19, 2004.

BLS. 2004b. Time-Use Survey—First Results Announced by BLS and Technical Note. *News.* U.S. Department of Labor, Washington, D.C., Sept. 14.

Brownson, R. C., and T. K. Boehmer. 2004. *Patterns and Trends in Physical Activity, Occupation, Transportation, Land Use, and Sedentary Behaviors.* Department of Community Health and Prevention Research Center, School of Public Health, St. Louis University. Prepared for the Committee on Physical Activity, Health, Transportation, and Land Use, June 25.

Bruno, L. C. 1993. *On the Move: A Chronology of Advances in Transportation.* Gale Research, Inc., Detroit, Mich.

BTS. 2003. *NHTS 2001 Highlights Report.* BTS03-05. U.S. Department of Transportation, Washington, D.C.

Carlino, G. A. 2000. From Centralization to Deconcentration: People and Jobs Spread Out. *Business Review,* Federal Reserve Bank of Philadelphia, Nov.–Dec., pp. 15–27.

Cutler, D. M., E. L. Glaser, and J. M. Shapiro. 2003. Why Have Americans Become More Obese? *Journal of Economic Perspectives,* Vol. 17, No. 3, Summer, pp. 93–118.

Dong, L., G. Block, and S. Mandel. 2004. Activities Contributing to Total Energy Expenditure in the United States: Results from the NHAPS Study. *International Journal of Behavioral Nutrition and Physical Activity,* Vol. 1, No. 4, Feb. 12.

DOT. 2001. *Summary Statistics on Demographic Characteristics and Total Travel 1969, 1977, 1983, 1990, and 1995 NPTS, and 2001 NHTS.* nhts.ornl.gov/2001/html_files/ trends_verb6.shtml. Accessed March 9, 2004.

EPA. 2003. *Travel and Environmental Implications of School Siting.* EPA-231-R-03-004. Washington, D.C.

Federal Register. 2000. Standards for Defining Metropolitan and Micropolitan Statistical Areas. Notice of Decision. Office of Management and Budget. Vol. 65, No. 249, Dec. 27, pp. 82227–82238.

Hu, P. S., and J. R. Young. 1999. *Summary of Travel Trends, 1995 Nationwide Personal Transportation Survey.* Federal Highway Administration, U.S. Department of Transportation, Dec.

IOM. 2004. *Preventing Childhood Obesity: Health in the Balance.* National Academies Press, Washington, D.C.

Jargowsky, P. A. 2003. *Stunning Progress, Hidden Problems: The Dramatic Decline of Concentrated Poverty in the 1990s.* Center on Urban and Metropolitan Policy, Brookings Institution, May.

Massey, D., and N. Denton. 1993. *American Apartheid: Segregation and the Making of the Underclass.* Harvard University Press, Cambridge, Mass.

Mieszkowski, P., and E. S. Mills. 1993. The Causes of Metropolitan Suburbanization. *Journal of Economic Perspectives,* Vol. 7, No. 3, pp. 137–147.

NRC. 1999. *Governance and Opportunity in Metropolitan America.* A. Altshuler, W. Morrill, H. Wolman, and F. Mitchell (eds.), National Academy Press, Washington, D.C.

Pucher, J., and J. I. Renne. 2003. Socioeconomics of Urban Travel: Evidence from the 2001 NHTS. *Transportation Quarterly,* Vol. 57, No. 3, Summer, pp. 49–77.

Robinson, J. P., and G. Godbey. 1999. *Time for Life: The Surprising Ways Americans Use Their Time,* 2nd ed. Pennsylvania State University Press, University Park.

TRB. 2002. *Special Report 269: The Relative Risks of School Travel: A National Perspective and Guidance for Local Community Risk Assessment.* National Research Council, Washington, D.C.

U.S. Bureau of the Census. 2002. *Racial and Ethnic Residential Segregation in the United States: 1980–2000.* U.S. Government Printing Office, Washington, D.C.

SUMMARY

Contextual Factors Affecting
Physical Activity

Recent national surveys report that Americans walk, and to a lesser extent cycle, primarily for exercise and recreation. However, reported levels of both activities fall short of recommended daily guidelines (i.e., 30 minutes per day of moderate-level physical activity on 5 or more days per week), a result confirmed by the public health surveys reviewed in Chapter 2. The barriers to meeting adequate physical activity levels include personal reasons (disabilities and other health impairments), concerns for safety and security, and time constraints and environmental impediments (long distances between destinations, limited travel choices).

From the perspective of environmental barriers, it is important to distinguish among different population groups and their geographic locations. Impediments to walking, cycling, and other forms of physical activity are likely to differ greatly among an inner-city neighborhood, a typical suburban development, and a remote rural community. Interventions to encourage greater physical activity should be tailored to reflect these differences, and the target populations should be segmented accordingly.

It is also important to distinguish among different types of physical activity in addressing environmental barriers. Americans appear to be interested and engaged in walking and cycling for recreation and, to a lesser extent, for local shopping. Interventions should reinforce these behaviors and provide opportunities for those who want to be physically active. Moreover, while the convenience and mobility of the car for commuting and regional shopping trips are not easily matched by walking or cycling, census data indicate that many Americans have convenient access to satisfactory neighborhood shopping, schools, and public transit, which provides numerous opportunities for using nonmotorized travel.

Opportunities to modify the built environment to make it more conducive to physical activity are numerous, but the ease or difficulty of such changes depends on the intervention. For example, overturning long-standing zoning and land use ordinances to increase development density and mixed land uses is likely to face formidable barriers that cannot easily be overcome. Bringing investment back to inner-city neighborhoods and creating safe environments with desirable destinations conducive to walking are long-term processes. More flexible and targeted approaches—such as context-sensitive design, special overlay districts, traffic calming measures, and community policing—are more likely to win support and can be implemented more rapidly. Construction of new buildings and developments also offers promising opportunities for creating more activity-friendly environments. To design effective policies and interventions, however, will require a more complete understanding of how the built environment facilitates or constrains physical activity, a topic investigated in the following two chapters.

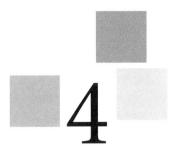

Contextual Factors Affecting Physical Activity

The preceding chapter documented many long-term trends in the way the U.S. population lives, works, and travels that have sharply reduced the physical demands of daily life. The persuasive scientific evidence on the importance of physical activity for health presents a challenge: to increase physical activity in a highly technological society with a built environment that is already in place and has evolved over a long period of time. This chapter explores the socio-economic and institutional context that has resulted in the current situation and holds the key to change. It starts with a discussion of the various factors that affect the individual's choices about engaging in physical activity. The chapter then turns to the institutional and regulatory forces behind the decisions of planners, engineers, developers, elected officials, and others over the years that have shaped the built environment in place today.

FACTORS AFFECTING INDIVIDUAL CHOICE

As discussed in Chapter 1 (Figure 1-1), physical activity behavior is influenced by both individual characteristics and the social environment. Whether an individual is physically active depends on demographic characteristics such as gender, age, and ethnic background, and on socioeconomic characteristics such as education and income level. It also depends on at least three other factors, the latter two of which are external to the individual: (*a*) attitudes, preferences, motivations, and skills related to the behavior; (*b*) opportunities or constraints that make the behavior easier or more difficult to perform; and (*c*) incentives or disincentives that encourage or discourage the desired behavior relative to competing activities. Each of these factors is discussed in turn in this section. Much of the discussion is based on self-reported survey data and focus groups. Relative to observational surveys, self-reported data often provide unreliable estimates because of problems with recall or the well-established tendency of survey respondents to give socially desirable rather than completely truthful answers (see Chapter 2). Results from focus groups cannot be generalized to the population at large. Nevertheless, self-reports and focus groups are the only way to obtain insight into attitudes and motivations that help explain behavior. This type of information is particularly important because the determinants of physical activity behavior are not well understood.

Socioeconomic Characteristics

The Behavioral Risk Factor Surveillance System (BRFSS) and the National Health Interview Survey (NHIS) have revealed that physical activity levels of U.S. adults decline with age and are lower among women, ethnic and racial minorities, those with less education and low income levels, the disabled, and those living in the southeastern region of the United States (see Chapter 2).[1] These results have been corroborated by numerous other studies.[2] For example, younger age is positively associated with physical activity, as are university education and higher income levels. Although comparisons by race are often obscured by socioeconomic variables, some studies have shown that ethnic minorities, particularly African American and Hispanic women, are less likely to adopt and maintain active lifestyles. Other personal barriers to walking

---

[1] The BRFSS is discussed in detail by Brownson and Boehmer (2004) and the NHIS by Barnes and Schoenborn (2003).

[2] See the commissioned paper by Loukaitou-Sideris (2004), which references several relevant studies on the effect of individual characteristics on the propensity to engage in physical activity.

and an active lifestyle cited in the literature include state of personal health and physical disability; lack of time, motivation, and energy; and lack of self-esteem. Further elaboration is not provided here because the committee has chosen to focus its discussion on physical activity behaviors linked with the built environment, such as nonmotorized travel and attitudes toward walking and cycling.

Attitudes, Preferences, Motivation, and Skills[3]

Several national surveys have been conducted in recent years to determine the public's attitudes toward walking and cycling, as well as the frequency and purpose of these behaviors. Two of the surveys were sponsored by organizations that advocate walking and cycling—the Surface Transportation Policy Project and America Bikes. They found positive attitudes among respondents toward both walking and cycling and strong support for investments that would make communities more friendly to these modes (BR&S 2003; America Bikes 2003).

A national survey of walking and cycling sponsored by the National Highway Traffic Safety Administration and the Bureau of Transportation Statistics (BTS) and administered by the Gallup Organization during summer 2002 found that 8 of 10 respondents aged 16 or older had taken at least one walk of 5 minutes or longer in the past 30 days; fewer than 30 percent, however, reported having ridden a bicycle at least once (DOT 2003). When asked the primary purpose for walking trips, respondents most commonly cited exercise or health reasons (27 percent), personal errands (17 percent), and recreation (15 percent). The primary purposes for cycling trips were recreation (26 percent) and exercise or health reasons (24 percent).[4] Survey results

---

[3] The following subsections draw heavily on the commissioned paper prepared for the committee by Kirby and Hollander (2004).

[4] Although only the primary trip purpose was recorded, the responses can be misleading. For example, the respondent may have indicated commuting to school or work as the primary trip purpose but may also have walked or cycled to work for exercise. Thus, there is likely to be overlap among some of these responses.

should be interpreted with caution because of low response rates.[5]

Another survey, conducted as part of the BTS monthly Omnibus Household Survey (BTS 2003), queried adults aged 18 and older about walking and cycling, among other forms of transportation, during 2001–2002.[6] [These results should also be interpreted with caution because of problems with response rates and sampling as detailed in a TRB report (2003).] Approximately 72 percent of those interviewed reported having walked, run, or jogged outside for 10 minutes or more at least once during the month prior to the survey (BTS 2003). Nearly 60 percent of those who walked, ran, or jogged (about 40 percent of all respondents) reported spending about 30 minutes on these activities an average of 13 days per month, as compared with the recommended minimum of 30 minutes per day of moderate-intensity activity on 5 or more days per week (see Chapter 2). Nearly 20 percent of respondents reported a longer duration of activity, but 40 percent reported no outside walking, running, or jogging (BTS 2003).[7] Only 16 percent of adult U.S. residents reported cycling outside during the month prior to the survey—spending just over 1 hour per day cycling on an average of 6 days per month (BTS 2002).

The Omnibus survey also inquired about the reasons for walking and cycling. Slightly more than three-quarters of those respondents who walked, ran, or jogged reported that they did so

---

[5] The survey was conducted by telephone and used a random sample of listed and unlisted numbers in the 50 states and the District of Columbia, which yielded 9,616 interviews with respondents aged 16 years or older, a 27 percent response rate. The results were then weighted to reflect the national population of this age group, with an estimated sampling error of about ±1.5 percentage points at the 95 percent confidence level.

[6] In 2000, BTS began a monthly national telephone survey to ascertain the public's satisfaction with the transportation system. Approximately 1,000 randomly selected households are telephoned each month, and the results are weighted to allow inferences about the U.S. population aged 18 or older. Periodically, questions are added for specific purposes, such as this survey of walking and cycling behavior. The walking survey was conducted from January to November 2002 and the cycling survey from October 2001 to September 2002.

[7] Nearly 30 percent of those who walked, ran, or jogged (20 percent of the total) reported spending an hour or more on these activities on about 13 days during a month.

primarily for exercise or recreation. Another 15 percent walked for personal errands, and only 7 percent to get to work or as part of their job (BTS 2003, 1).[8] Similarly, the primary reasons for cycling were for recreation (54 percent) or exercise (33 percent); only 6 percent reported commuting by bicycle to get to school or work or as part of their job (BTS 2002).

In sum, the surveys indicate that walking is more prevalent than cycling, but reported levels of walking appear to fall short of recommended daily guidelines. To the extent that Americans report walking and cycling, the primary reasons appear to be for exercise and recreation. These results correspond with the behavioral data from public health surveys discussed in the previous chapter showing a trend toward increased leisure-time physical activity.

Market research has also been conducted to probe the reasons for engaging in physical activity. Several studies cited by Kirby and Hollander (2004)[9] found that adults' dominant beliefs about moderate physical activity were that it results in feeling better or more energetic, helps reduce stress, and improves physical condition (e.g., feeling less out of breath, stronger). Focus groups with older Americans revealed similar beliefs.[10] Notably absent from the survey and focus group results is any mention of the longer-term benefits of physical activity identified by the health community and summarized in Chapter 2, such as disease prevention. The positive health effects of physical activity may have been assumed by the survey and focus group respondents, but the results may also reflect the value placed by many people on more immediate benefits, such as those enumerated above. In any event, the market research

---

[8] As with the Gallup surveys, the respondents were asked their primary trip purpose. However, there can be an overlap in the responses between travel for exercise and for utilitarian purposes.

[9] Fridinger et al. 1996; Collette et al. 1994; Wankel and Mummery 1993; Brown 1992; Kotler et al. 2002.

[10] For midlife adults, the focus groups revealed that physical activity was perceived as a way to fight aging, to continue to look good, and to cope with a changing life. Older preretired adults mentioned having more energy, prolonging an active life, and protecting their quality of life as benefits of physical activity. Retired adults said they engaged in physical activity to ensure a high quality of life, maintain connections in the community, and maintain everyday functions and independence (Sloan 2001 in Kirby and Hollander 2004).

results underscore the importance of understanding the beliefs and attitudes of those whose behavior one wishes to reinforce or change. As marketers are well aware, beliefs and attitudes are likely to differ across subpopulations. For example, a single mother holding two jobs is likely to be motivated to become more physically active by information showing how physical activity can be fit into her busy daily routine, whereas a teenager is likely to be more motivated by information that physical activity will make her more fit and attractive. Thus, tailoring interventions to specific groups is likely to prove more effective than delivering mass messages about the benefits of being physically active.

Finally, while beliefs, attitudes, and preferences have a role in determining a person's physical activity habits, cognitive and behavioral factors come into play as well. To become more physically active, for example, individuals can self-monitor the target behavior, learn how to set realistic and achievable goals, monitor progress toward those goals, identify barriers to achieving the goals, use problem-solving techniques to overcome those barriers, and identify and use peer and family social support to help achieve lasting behavioral change. Interventions using these methods, which are based on psychosocial theories and models such as social cognitive theory and motivational readiness, have been applied successfully in randomized, controlled clinical trials to evaluate methods of helping sedentary adults become more active (Kohl et al. 1998; King et al. 1998; Dunn et al. 1999). The committee is unaware, however, of published reports in which cognitive and behavioral interventions have been incorporated into designs that also encompass environmental and socio-economic factors.

Opportunities and Constraints

The results of the surveys reviewed in the previous section and those of other large health surveys presented in Chapter 2 indicate that the majority of Americans are not acting sufficiently on their inclinations to meet recommended levels of total daily physical activity. Personal motivation is one likely explanation, but it is instructive to examine other possible factors—real or perceived—that may be preventing the desired behavior, with particular attention to the built environment as a potential barrier. It should be noted that, although walking and cycling are discussed together here, they generally involve different infrastructure and user characteristics. For example, in urban areas, cycling typically is forbidden on sidewalks and confined to certain streets or bicycle lanes that share the right-of-way with automobiles. Cycling on pedestrian paths can pose a danger for those who are walking. These differences should be kept in mind in interpreting survey results. For example, these differences are likely to make cyclists more concerned with infrastructure facilities for safety.

The Gallup survey discussed above revealed that the primary reasons for not walking or cycling were personal (disabilities or other health impairments), weather- or time-related, or equipment-related (did not own or have access to a bicycle) (DOT 2003). Environmental factors (no safe place to ride or walk) were mentioned by only a small fraction of respondents (approximately 3 percent) (DOT 2003). Three of four adults reported being "very" or "somewhat satisfied" with the design of their communities for pedestrian safety. Nevertheless, when asked to recommend changes in their communities, presumably to make walking safer, about one-third of those polled suggested providing pedestrian facilities, such as sidewalks, traffic signals, lighting, and crosswalks. Satisfaction with the cycling environment was considerably lower. Only half of those polled were "very" or "somewhat satisfied" with their communities' designs for cycling safety. Nearly one-half of all respondents recommended new bicycle facilities, such as bicycle trails, paths, lanes, racks, traffic signals, lighting, and crosswalks. The survey results suggest that, even for those favorably disposed to walking and cycling, changes to the physical environment that would enhance the safety and ease of engaging in these activities could make a difference.

Results of other surveys suggest that environmental factors may play a more dominant role depending on the activity—for example, transporting children to school. As noted earlier, the private vehicle has become the primary mode of school travel (Dellinger and Staunton 2002). Long distances, dangerous traffic, and crime have been mentioned as the main barriers to children walking and cycling more to school (Dellinger and Staunton 2002; BR&S 2003).[11] In fact, children (aged 5 to 18) of parents who reported no barriers [16 percent of all respondents to the Centers for Disease Control and Prevention's (CDC's) HealthStyles Survey reported by Dellinger and Staunton] were six times more likely to walk or bicycle to school than those whose parents cited one or more barriers.

Interventions to mitigate such barriers can be effective. For example, the California Safe Routes to School Program has provided more than $40 million to municipalities and counties to improve the safety and viability of walking and cycling to school. Typical projects include sidewalk construction and improvements, pedestrian and bicycle crossings, and traffic controls to improve the safety of street crossings (Boarnet 2004). A before-and-after evaluation of projects associated with 10 schools across the state found that walking and cycling had increased, with larger effects if the project was along the child's usual route to school (Boarnet et al. 2004).[12] The Marin County Safe Routes to School Program is a good example of a comprehensive approach to reducing barriers for children walking and cycling to school that appears to be working (see Box 4-1).

Constraints and barriers to physical activity are perhaps best illustrated in those low-income neighborhoods where crime, disinvestment, and isolation can be major deterrents to walking and cycling for many residents. Low-income urban populations

---

[11] The HealthStyles 1999 Survey, analyzed by CDC and reported by Dellinger and Staunton (2002), found that major reported barriers to walking and cycling to school included long distances (55 percent), traffic danger (40 percent), adverse weather conditions (24 percent), and crime (18 percent). The BR&S 2003 survey found distance to be the primary barrier (mentioned by 66 percent), followed by traffic danger (17 percent), fear of child being abducted (16 percent), inconvenience (15 percent), and neighborhood crime (15 percent). For both surveys, multiple responses were accepted; hence the percentages do not add up to 100.

[12] Survey respondents reported an increase of 10.5 percent in walking and cycling to school associated with the construction improvements. A slightly higher percentage—15.4 percent—was reported if the improvements were along the child's usual route to school.

BOX 4-1

The Marin County, California, Safe Routes to School Program

The Safe Routes to School Program in Marin County is one of the programs funded by the California Safe Routes to School Program. Marin County has established a grassroots program that is getting more children to walk and bicycle to school.

Program components include mapping of routes and infrastructure improvements to improve access to schools by walking or bicycling, special events and contest promotions, new concepts such as "walking school buses" and "bike trains" to generate and maintain the interest of the community, and a well-integrated communication and promotion strategy. Safe Routes task forces collaborate with public works and law enforcement staff to develop and implement an improvement plan, apply for funding, and effect improvements such as crosswalks and signage to make it easier and more convenient to walk and cycle to school. The California headquarters for the Safe Routes to School Program also provides materials, tips, and tools for community volunteers and organizations. These include a walkability checklist, sample letters to parents in 13 languages, a "guide to success" with instructions on how to create a walking school bus and a bike train, and a guide on how to create safe drop-off points for children walking to school (see www.cawalktoschool.com/dropoff_zones.php). In addition, the California headquarters partners with the state health department's injury control center to give its safety messages even more credibility with parents.

Most important, the program appears to be working. At the second-year mark of the commencement of the program in Marin County, 15 participating public schools reported an increase in walking (64 percent), bicycling (114 percent), and carpooling (91 percent) and a decrease in private vehicles carrying only one student (39 percent) (Staunton et al. 2003).

SOURCE: Kirby and Hollander 2004.

exhibit the highest levels of walking and bus transit use[13] for utilitarian travel out of necessity (Pucher and Renne 2003), but they engage in much less discretionary physical activity than other groups (see Chapter 2). Interventions such as the Sisters Together Program (see Box 4-2), which attempt to address issues of regaining control over one's environment (e.g., safe walk routes) and combating isolation (e.g., walking buddies), may help overcome barriers to recreational physical activity for some low-income urban populations. Not all low- or moderate-income neighborhoods are affected by fears of crime, however. Physical inactivity of their residents must derive from other causes.

Concern for personal safety can also play a role in the use of pathways for walking and jogging in urban and regional parks. Surveys and focus groups have shown that adults, particularly older adults and female minorities, perceive unsafe footpaths and other recreational areas for exercise as deterrents to walking and other physical activity (Hahn and Craythorn 1994; King et al. 2000; Booth et al. 2000).

Crime and deteriorated neighborhoods are less likely to be an issue in rural settings, where natural scenery (open fields) and lightly traveled rural roads provide opportunities for walking and cycling. For the rural poor, however, isolation and long distances between destinations may limit these activities (Brownson et al. 2000 in Kirby and Hollander 2004).

Providing opportunities for walking and cycling may not be sufficient to change behavior, however, particularly for certain types of travel, such as commuting. Time constraints, long distances between destinations, and the mobility afforded by the automobile make traveling by personal vehicle the preferred option for many commuters. A recent study of commuting behavior in three neighborhoods in the San Francisco Bay Area—one urban and two suburban—attempted to separate the effects of household location preferences from the spatial characteristics of residential neighbor-

---

[13] As noted earlier, transit, particularly bus transit, requires some walking to access the bus stop. Rail transit can also induce walking and cycling, but in suburban locations, park-and-ride facilities make driving an option.

BOX 4-2

The Sisters Together Program

This obesity prevention pilot program supported by the National Institutes of Health (NIH) and the National Institute of Diabetes and Digestive and Kidney Diseases (www.niddk.nih.gov/health/nutrit/pdf/SisPrmGuide2.pdf) began by targeting young black women in three inner-city neighborhoods of Boston. The campaign focused on creating positive messages to generate normative change and involving existing community programs to build sustainability.

The Sisters Together initiative developed a coalition of programs and people in the community, targeting both healthy eating and moving more (www.hsph.harvard.edu/sisterstogether/move.html). In an effort to suggest activities that would resonate with their target audiences, program staff developed tips on dancing, not just walking: "Turn on your favorite music and dance to three songs a day three times a week. It gets your heart pumping, your body moving, and your mind feeling great." A web page and brochure provided safe walking routes around the city. Radio public service announcements offered women a chance to sign up for a neighborhood walking group if they came to a 2-mile warm-up walking event. Making it easier for women to locate a walking buddy helped promote a positive social norm with regard to walking. The program's *Why Walk* cites the top three benefits of walking validated by research—"Walking will . . . give you more energy, make you feel good, and help you relax."

A traditional method—the bounce-back card—was used to obtain feedback from the target audience and partners on how the program was working and what could be improved. Community partners were engaged to be the sustaining force behind the program once NIH funding for the pilot project ended. Rudd et al. (1999) describe the community development model employed in this project, but no longer-term evaluation data could be located.

SOURCE: Kirby and Hollander 2004.

hoods that help shape travel patterns (Schwanen and Mokhtarian 2004). The researchers found that, even after controlling for socio-demographic characteristics, mobility limitations, personality and lifestyle types, and travel attitudes, suburban-minded residents of the urban neighborhood (i.e., urban dwellers who preferred lower-density environments) commuted by private vehicle far more than their urban-minded neighbors (those who preferred higher-density environments such as the one in which they lived). Similarly, urban-minded suburban dwellers commuted by car about as often as their suburban-minded neighbors. However, the differences in commuting behavior across neighborhoods were greater than those within neighborhoods, which indicates that neighborhood structure itself has an autonomous effect on travel choices. Commuting by personal vehicle strongly prevails in suburban neighborhoods in which residents have fewer mode choices, longer distances to travel, and lifestyle preferences for low-density living. In urban neighborhoods where densities are higher, travel distances are often shorter, and travel options are greater, transit achieves a higher commute mode share than in suburban neighborhoods (Schwanen and Mokhtarian 2004).

Incentives and Disincentives

Lowering the cost of a desired behavior and raising the price of an undesired behavior can be an effective strategy for motivating behavior change. The choice to walk, bicycle, or combine either with transit may require such incentives and disincentives. For example, a combination of providing transit fare subsidies through the workplace and either cashing out[14] or raising parking fees could help level the playing field between driving and taking transit and encourage greater transit use (Shoup 1994; Shoup 1997).[15] (Of course, the

---

[14] "Cashing out" refers to employers offering employees the cash equivalent of any employee parking subsidy. The idea is that at least some commuters who previously drove alone to work might take the cash and choose an alternative mode, such as ridesharing (Shoup 1997).

[15] These strategies, however, are complex. Care must be taken to consider distributional issues, for example, in their implementation. A more detailed discussion of equity issues is given in *Special Report 242* (TRB 1994).

workplace must be accessible to transit for the employee to take advantage of the transit fare subsidy.)

In addition to monetary incentives, such strategies as reducing the time cost of physical activity—making it easier and more convenient to be physically active—can be effective. In the previously cited national survey conducted by BR&S on Americans' attitudes toward walking, inconvenience (destinations being too far) and time were the primary reasons cited for not walking more (BR&S 2003). Likewise, a community intervention in Wheeling, West Virginia, targeting sedentary adults aged 50 to 65 found that time and schedule were the major stated deterrents to being physically active (see Box 4-3) (Reger et al. 2002 in Kirby and Hollander 2004). With the tagline "Isn't it time you started walking?" the intervention attempted to make the case that walking is an activity easily accommodated and integrated into one's daily routine. Similarly, one of CDC's earliest campaigns to promote the benefits of moderate physical activity—with the slogan "Ready, Set, It's Everywhere You Go"—sought to underscore that moderate-intensity activities could easily be part of the daily routine (see Box 4-4) (Kirby and Hollander 2004). Lack of evaluation of such projects for their effects on physical activity levels, however, makes it impossible to predict the benefits of such approaches.

Improving access by shortening distances between destinations is more difficult to address. Such a strategy requires moving one's residence or employment or both, or locating facilities in closer proximity to one another—a topic discussed in the following section.

To create incentives for physical activity, one must also consider the competition for the desired behavior. For example, a competitor for engaging in recreational physical activity might be watching television (Kirby and Hollander 2004), although this need not be the case. Many individuals watch television, or could be encouraged to do so, as they walk a treadmill either in their homes or at sports clubs. Another, more challenging competitor is the car, particularly for utilitarian physical activity. As Schwanen and Mokhtarian (2004) found, improving nonautomobile mode choice options can help encourage transit use and related walking, but these modes

BOX 4-3

Wheeling, Virginia, Intervention
for Sedentary Adults Aged 50–65

The work of Reger et al. (2002) is a good example of using marketing principles to design a behavior change effort. First, the researchers decided on a specific behavior—walking—for a specific target audience—sedentary adults aged 50 to 65 in Wheeling, West Virginia.

Initially, most of the programmatic effort was focused on promotion and price variables. Formative research had found that sedentary and irregularly active people and regular walkers share similar attitudes and normative beliefs but exhibit strong differences related to their perceived control over time and scheduling. The major "price" of walking for the sedentary adult was "time." Thus, the ensuing promotional strategy was focused on perceived control issues and positioned walking as an activity that was easy to accommodate and integrate into one's daily routine. A pithy tagline was developed to address the time issue: "Isn't it time you started walking?"

The formative research also identified optimal promotional channels for reaching the intended audience. A combination of paid advertisements on television and radio and in newspapers was developed. In addition, non–mass media channels were tapped, such as the Wheeling Medical Society, physician prescriptions, work site wellness challenges, and community walking events. After initial campaign efforts, the researchers remained in contact with community participants, who suggested various improvements in community walking facilities. The mayor was engaged; a community task force was established; and collaboration with the National Park Service, the state Department of Transportation, and a local Rails-to-Trails group was initiated.

The following quotation illustrates the power of addressing perceived behavioral control:

> My biggest surprise about walking was the fact that I actually could do it. When my brother found out how far I was going he talked me into racing. I didn't think I could do it, but luckily I won my first race and from then on I was hooked. I loved the people, the atmosphere, and the challenge.

SOURCE: Kirby and Hollander 2004.

BOX 4-4

CDC's "Ready, Set, It's Everywhere You Go" Campaign

CDC launched one of the earliest campaigns to encourage moderate physical activity as opposed to "exercise," which had a more high-intensity, time-demanding connotation. CDC's "Ready, Set, It's Everywhere You Go" campaign relied mainly on communication techniques to introduce the notion of moderate-intensity activity that could be part of an adult's routine daily life. Formative research was conducted to validate audience segmentation and develop materials and promotional messages.

CDC produced a marketing kit for use by community-based organizations in their local efforts. It comprised three parts: (*a*) marketing strategies for physical activity, (*b*) ways to work with the media, and (*c*) the development of physical activity programs and events. The kit included a colorful poster and print ad emphasizing that people can be active doing routine activities such as yard work and walking the dog. The kit was designed to help health professionals and community-based organizations identify adults who wanted to become physically active and reach them with accurate and positive messages that had been tested with the same target audience. Target audiences specifically wanted materials that were family-friendly and conveyed the idea of having fun and being energetic.

By analyzing market research data and conducting focus groups and interviews, CDC developed a detailed picture of the intended audience. Research revealed that the majority of the intended audience was 18 to 45 years old, educated, middle-income, and female. Since 71 percent were married, 74 percent were employed, and 58 percent had live-in children, it was not surprising that these adults reported having little time for themselves after meeting their household, job, and family demands. Few of them considered themselves rugged or athletic; rather, they described themselves as interesting, friendly, caring, mature, fun, smart, honest, and content. As a whole, the target group members reported that they did not enjoy vigorous

(continued)

BOX 4-4 (*continued*)

"exercise." However, they did view "physical activity" as fun and enjoyable and were pleased to learn that it is important to their health and well-being. Participants believed that internal motivation, pleasant and manageable activities, support from family and friends, and convenience would help them become more physically active.

A variety of other barriers stood in the way of physical activity. Participants in the research cited such barriers as long work hours, being tired at the end of the day, lack of confidence in their athletic ability, and family priorities. Program planners reasoned that helping people understand that physical activity is "everywhere" they go and easy to do could help them become more active. The "Ready, Set, It's Everywhere You Go" materials, community kit, radio spots, and posters were audience tested—an important step in formative evaluation for marketing. The project has not been evaluated for its impact on changing behavior related to physical activity or healthy eating, however.

SOURCE: Kirby and Hollander 2004.

cannot always compete with the mobility and convenience afforded by the personal vehicle. Fortunately, total levels of physical activity matter, not whether an individual drives rather than walks or cycles to work, and even modest increases in total physical activity levels can have a positive effect on health (see Chapter 2). Nevertheless, it must be acknowledged that some individuals may view physical activity—even in small amounts—as unpleasant.

INSTITUTIONAL AND REGULATORY CONTEXT

Whereas the previous section examined the demand for physical activity, this section looks at the supply side of the link between the built environment and physical activity. Specifically, it examines the institutional and regulatory arrangements and policies that, over time, have created the built environment in place today.[16]

Zoning and Land Use Ordinances

In the United States, local governments are responsible for developing comprehensive plans and establishing land use regulations that determine how a community will develop. The authority to create zoning and subdivision controls and building regulations, which have the force of law, is a powerful tool in establishing the design requirements and physical context of a community's development. Most zoning regulations and subdivision controls regulate two factors thought to be closely linked to a community's walkability and bikeability—development densities and mixing of land uses.

Zoning was introduced by urban reformers in the United States in the early twentieth century to help alleviate the impacts of urban overcrowding on disease and illness. New York's Zoning Ordinance of 1916—the first enacted in the nation—was created for the express purpose of limiting development densities and thereby improving public health (Jurgensmeyer and Roberts 1998 in Meyer and Dumbaugh 2004). Early zoning regulations prohibited mixing of land uses to segregate those that would be incompatible, such as residential and high-polluting industrial uses. As they evolved, zoning laws also operated to reinforce economic and racial separation. Exclusionary zoning in wealthier communities restricted certain types of development, such as multifamily housing construction, and established stringent standards, such as minimum lot sizes or housing square footage, that had the effect of keeping housing prices high and thus excluding lower-income families (NRC 1999). Once such zoning limits were in place, they tended to be reinforcing. Households that moved to a community with single-family zoning viewed efforts to incorporate more affordable multifamily housing as a threat to their property values (Fischel 1999 in NRC 1999).

---

[16] The following subsections draw heavily on the commissioned paper prepared for the committee by Meyer and Dumbaugh (2004).

Municipal street designs and zoning requirements regarding parking have also had an important impact on the development of communities. Early municipal street designs incorporated in guidelines issued by the U.S. Federal Housing Administration in 1935 recommended that residential streets be designed to "discourage through traffic, have a minimum paved width of 24 feet, use cul-de-sacs[17] as much as possible, and avoid excessive planting in the front yards to have a 'more pleasing and unified effect along the street' " (FHA 1935). Municipal street design standards were also developed to take into account requirements for providing emergency services. Wide streets were believed necessary to accommodate the worst-case scenario—two high-rise ladder trucks jockeying for position on a dead-end street (Duany et al. 2000 in Meyer and Dumbaugh 2004).

Most community zoning codes require that a minimum number of parking spaces be provided per unit or per 1,000 square feet to accommodate the maximum demand for parking (Meyer and Dumbaugh 2004). In most cases, this number is greater than what is needed to handle "normal" demand and results in an oversupply of parking, particularly in suburban areas.

Taken together, zoning and land use controls can make it difficult to provide many of the characteristics associated with walkable and bikeable communities today (Meyer and Dumbaugh 2004). For example, low-density development often results in long distances between destinations, and research suggests that walking and cycling are highly sensitive to distance as compared with automobile travel, particularly travel for utilitarian purposes. Walking speeds are about 3 miles per hour (mph), and average bicycle speeds are about

---

[17] A cul-de-sac is a street, lane, or passage closed at one end. Its primary use, which is encouraged by traffic engineering and subdivision standards, has been to control through traffic in residential developments (Southworth and Ben-Joseph 2004). The cul-de-sac and its close cousin—the longer-loop street with two access points—have been criticized by the new urbanists for their lack of connectedness and their adverse effect on congestion, since all traffic must enter and exit the development through a limited number of access points. On the other hand, one could argue that families who live on cul-de-sacs feel safer letting their children play outdoors than those who live on through streets. And in some communities, connections to bicycle paths and greenbelt systems exist.

8 mph, depending on topography. Some planners suggest that walkable communities should have destinations within roughly ¼ to ½ mile of the point of origin (Seneviratne 1985). Bicycle destinations can be located slightly farther—2 to 3 miles from the point of origin (Meyer and Dumbaugh 2004). These guidelines are simply rules of thumb—individuals may well be willing to walk and cycle longer distances—but they underscore the competition posed by faster transport modes.

Separation of land uses also tends to increase the distances between destinations and creates a monotonous environment that may not be conducive to walking or cycling. In today's economy, the rationale for separating land uses is less compelling; many service-related work places are compatible with residential uses. Minimum parking requirements accommodate driving to most destinations and take up space that could be used for neighborhood amenities, such as parks and green spaces. Finally, wide residential streets with long straight sight lines and few trees contribute to vehicle speeding, creating a potentially dangerous environment for pedestrians and cyclists (Meyer and Dumbaugh 2004).

Urban Design Features

Design features are also thought to affect the form of community development and travel choices. Such features refer to both the aesthetic appeal and the function of buildings, streetscapes, and public spaces, which can be designed in ways that can encourage walking and transit use, particularly in the neighborhood, but also around work sites. Table 4-1 lists five such urban design features—density of development, land use mix, street connectivity, street scale, and aesthetic qualities—and describes how they can be measured.

The writings of Jane Jacobs in the 1960s (Jacobs 1961) and Kenneth Jackson in the 1980s (Jackson 1985) critiqued the loss of neighborhood scale and community life in the automobile-dependent suburbs created largely after World War II. Whyte and Appleyard's studies of public spaces and livable streets in the early 1980s (Whyte 1980; Appleyard 1981) and architect Peter

TABLE 4-1   Examples of Design Features of the Built Environment

Design Element	Description and Possible Measures
Density	The amount of activity found in an area—usually defined as population, employment, or building square footage per unit of area and measured as people per acre or jobs per square mile. Floor–area ratio, the ratio between the floor space in a building and the size of the parcel on which the building sits, is another density measure.
Land use mix	The relative proximity of different land uses (e.g., homes, stores, offices, parks) within a given area—no standard measure.
Street connectivity	The directness and availability of alternative routes from one point to another within a street network—measured by the number of intersections per square mile, average block length, and so forth.
Street scale	The three-dimensional space along a street as bounded by buildings or other features—typically described as "human-scale" or "automobile-scale"—measured by the average building setback or by the ratio between building heights and street widths.
Aesthetic qualities	The qualities that contribute to the attractiveness or appeal of a place, such as the design of buildings (size and orientation of windows), landscaping, lighting and benches—the most intangible of the design features—more often described than measured.

SOURCE: Adapted from Handy et al. 2002, 66.

Calthorpe's vision of more walkable and livable communities (Calthorpe 1993) gave rise to a set of design concepts collectively known as the "new urbanism." The movement emerged in the late 1980s through architects who designed smaller, people-oriented communities with a small-town feel and a village scale. The goal was to establish a sense of community—often missing in newly developed neighborhoods—by creating human-scale housing and streets, mixing land uses, providing vibrant public spaces, and getting people out of their cars (Boarnet and Crane 2001). New-urbanist developments emphasize such design elements as front porches, sidewalks, and common public spaces as gathering places for community activities.

The claim is made that walking will increase if the activities of daily living (e.g., parks, neighborhood shopping) are within walking distance and linked to where people live and work by an inter-connected network of streets, sidewalks, and paths (Handy et al. 2002). These goals can be achieved by straightening of streets to improve connectivity (i.e., use of grid street patterns), "calming" of traffic, more compact land uses with a diversity of destinations, and inviting street environments with amenities such as street furniture and plantings (Boarnet and Crane 2001). Transit use should also increase with more compact land use and clustering of shopping and housing near rail or bus nodes. The evidence supporting the effects of urban design features on walking, including walking to access transit facilities, is reviewed in the paper by Handy commissioned for this study (Handy 2004) and summarized in Chapter 6.

Developers' Response[18]

Private developers and lenders are ultimately responsible for the development and construction of local residences and commercial facilities. Recent surveys (Levine and Inam 2004; Smith-Heimer and Golem 2001 in Kirby and Hollander 2004) have revealed that real estate developers perceive considerable market interest in walkable communities and support developments with greater density and more mixed uses than regulations allow, particularly in inner-suburban areas. A panel discussion with California developers yielded evidence of good market support for transit-oriented development projects that involve mixed-use development near transit stations (Smith-Heimer and Golem 2001).

In view of these findings, why are there not more walking- and cycling-friendly developments—often called neotraditional or new-urbanist developments—and transit-oriented development projects in response to market demand, particularly since such developments are in short supply? Levine and Inam (2004) suggest that a large majority of developers perceive local zoning controls and the related costs of pursuing variances as the primary obstacles to neotraditional developments. For example, among developers

---

[18] This discussion of real estate developers also draws on the commissioned paper by Kirby and Hollander (2004).

who proposed neotraditional developments for which variances were granted, the density was reduced by the community planning process for approximately 80 percent, mixed-use characteristics were reduced for nearly 50 percent, the housing types were changed for nearly 30 percent, the share of mixed-use development was changed for one-third, and changes were made in pedestrian or transit orientation for nearly 20 percent (Levine and Inam 2004). Other surveys have revealed that public resistance to densification and neighborhood opposition to mixed-use development are significant barriers to neotraditional projects (Logan et al. 2001 in Kirby and Hollander 2004). These findings indicate that, when faced with accepting higher densities or mixed-use development—changes that may be perceived as negatively affecting property values—not all consumers are as supportive of more walking-, cycling-, and transit-friendly communities as their survey responses would suggest.

Financial institutions can also be a barrier. Despite some developers' perception that neotraditional developments can be profitable and the findings of studies confirming that this is in fact the case (Eppli and Tu 1999 in Kirby and Hollander 2004),[19] institutional lenders are risk averse. Typically, they look for projects that are compatible with other developments in the local market (i.e., that meet local zoning and subdivision controls). Financing of mixed-use developments can be particularly problematic because many lenders have experience in dealing with only one type of development (Meyer and Dumbaugh 2004; Kirby and

---

[19] Eppli and Tu (1999) examined neotraditional developments from a housing market perspective. They compared sales transactions and characteristics of homes in four regionally diverse new-urbanist developments with those of homes in nearby conventional neighborhoods. Properties in Kentlands, a new-urbanist development, were found to be selling for $30,000 to $40,000 more, on average, than homes in the surrounding conventional suburbs, even after controlling for site traits, housing characteristics, unit quality, neighborhood, and other market factors. In view of survey data revealing positive attitudes toward walking and the barriers posed by distance, inconvenience, and time constraints, it would appear that developments such as Kentlands could motivate and support increases in neighborhood walking and cycling. The fact that residents appear to be willing to pay a premium for living in such a community should hold some appeal for real estate developers.

Hollander 2004). An informal survey of institutional lenders in the Atlanta, Seattle, and Boston markets conducted by Meyer and Dumbaugh (2004), for example, revealed that lenders are not averse to neotraditional developments as long as such developments are not expressly prohibited by local zoning and are not the first such development in an area. The presence of profitable existing neotraditional developments in a local market and evidence of other public and private investment in a transit-oriented development, of course, increase the acceptability of similar new projects (Smith-Heimer and Golem 2001).

Relaxing zoning and financing barriers to enable more neotraditional development for those who would like to locate in such communities would require changes on many fronts—not the least of which would be to educate the public, elected officials, and the real estate community in how these communities can work and be implemented. The more it can be shown that such communities can be profitable and not reduce surrounding property values, the more acceptable they will become (Meyer and Dumbaugh 2004). In addition, instead of overturning long-standing zoning regulations and ordinances, it may be easier to win support through more targeted approaches, such as overlay districts[20] and incentives (Meyer and Dumbaugh 2004; see Box 4-5 for two examples).

School Design and Location

Decisions about school design and location are largely independent of the processes that drive other forms of community development. Planning for educational facilities is the responsibility of local school boards, which are typically composed of elected representatives. Because nearly all school boards are semiautonomous, they—not local governments that have a strong interest in the

---

[20] Overlay districts are a planning tool providing for special zoning requirements that are an exception to the underlying zoning and are tailored to the characteristics of a particular area (e.g., special architectural character) or complementary to a particular public policy (e.g., higher-density building near rail transit stations).

BOX 4-5

Two Approaches to Relaxation
of Zoning Regulations and Controls

Overlay districts. Changing a community's land use zoning is often a difficult political undertaking. One of the approaches used to provide a higher level of urban design while maintaining the underlying zoning is to use overlay zones targeting specific development characteristics. A good example is Portland, Oregon's, Light Rail Transit Station Zone (Portland Metro 2000). This overlay zone "allows for more intense and efficient use of land at increased densities for the mutual reinforcement of public investments and private development. Uses and development are regulated to create a more intense built-up environment, oriented to pedestrians, and ensuring a density and intensity that is transit supportive." Actions include prohibition of parking garages within a specified distance of a station, a 50 percent reduction in the minimum number of parking spaces required within 500 feet of a light rail alignment, and the requirement of a high level of streetscape landscaping.

Neotraditional development incentives. Restructuring long-standing land use ordinances that have been the basic approach to community development is also difficult. A more appealing approach for encouraging neotraditional development and use of nonmotorized transportation is to provide incentives to both developers and communities. For example, in specified districts, developers could receive income tax credits for certain types of development, reductions in permit fees and other procedural requirements, and relaxation of other zoning requirements that might save the developer money. Regional planning agencies could reward communities that provided approvals for neotraditional developments. In the San Francisco Bay Area, for example, the metropolitan planning organization provides a certain amount of money to a community for every bedroom constructed within a certain distance of a transit station. These funds can be used by the community for any purpose. By using incentives, policy makers participate in the development market, but not in the traditional regulatory way.

SOURCE: Meyer and Dumbaugh 2004.

overall development of a community—make decisions about school design and location.

The trend in school design has been to develop bigger schools to lower costs through economies of scale. The large land requirements recommended by the standards-setting organization for school facilities[21] make incorporating these schools into existing communities difficult. The trend is to locate the facilities on large suburban tracts, which necessitates driving or busing students from surrounding communities. Because local school boards are responsible only for on-site circulation and not for access from the surrounding street network, means of accommodating walking and cycling to school are rarely planned as part of a school construction project. Similarly, school bus routes and safe access to bus stops are under the purview of local school boards; little coordination with local community planners is involved (Meyer and Dumbaugh 2004).

Some states and communities have begun to reevaluate the desirability of requirements that encourage the building of large new school campuses (EPA 2003). For example, South Carolina recently eliminated state-mandated acreage requirements for new schools that may make it easier for existing schools to be renovated. Neighborhood school initiatives in Wisconsin and Minnesota have resulted in retaining many elementary schools within walkable neighborhoods.

More coordination between local school boards and local government planners could help in addressing issues of school access and optimum school location. At a minimum, initiatives such as the previously discussed Safe Routes to School Program could help encourage more walking and cycling to school or walking to school bus stops.

Modeling of Transportation Needs

All major metropolitan areas are required by the federally supported planning process to have a regional transportation model

---

[21] A professional organization, the Council for Educational Facilities Planners International, provides guidance on school design and construction.

for analyzing network investment needs and alternatives (Meyer and Dumbaugh 2004). These models provide a very aggregate picture of regional travel and were not intended to handle the level of detail required to analyze or predict pedestrian or cycling trips. Major roads, such as freeways and arterials, are represented by network links in the models, but most local roads where pedestrians walk and bicyclists ride are not. Many walking and cycling trips are relatively short in distance, occurring within a traffic analysis zone. Statistical averages are normally used to represent intrazonal travel. This can understate the impact of mixing land uses or improving pedestrian ways within a city block in promoting walking because averages ignore any variation around the mean. Overall, regional transportation models generally do a poor job of representing non-motorized travel, which can understate the potential role of pedestrian facilities and bicycle paths as well as land use strategies in promoting walking and cycling trips (Meyer and Dumbaugh 2004).

The typical regional transportation forecasting model consists of four major steps: trip generation, trip distribution, mode choice, and trip assignment. The first step, trip generation, is a function of exogenously determined demographic patterns and economic activity in a region. The remaining three steps, which are followed sequentially, simply allocate trips among alternative destinations in trip distribution, alternative travel modes in mode choice, and alternative highway (and transit if appropriate) routes in trip assignment (TRB 1995). Trip assignment is based primarily on minimizing travel time through an iterative process that feeds back to mode choice, and sometimes to trip distribution, in an effort to equate initial with final travel time estimates. The outputs of the model are vehicle and passenger volumes on highway and transit routes, respectively.

The recent interest in policies supporting pedestrian and bicycle travel has led some metropolitan areas, such as Portland, Oregon, and the San Francisco Bay Area, to make advances in incorporating pedestrian and bicycle travel into their transportation models. They are still the exception rather than the norm, however. Furthermore, few metropolitan areas have integrated land use and travel demand models, so that the effects of changes in urban form and design on travel behavior cannot be determined (Meyer and Dumbaugh 2004).

Models are important inputs to policy makers, but they represent only one element in the policy process. European cities typically have better bicycle and pedestrian facilities than most of their U.S. counterparts, but this is not an outcome of better models. Other policies, such as higher gasoline prices that discourage automobile travel, have likely played a far greater role in investment in nonmotorized facilities.

Roadway Infrastructure Design

A highly standardized approach to roadway infrastructure design has also played a major role in determining the design and development of communities (Meyer and Dumbaugh 2004). The design manuals used by highway and traffic engineers—the "Green Book" of the American Association of State Highway and Transportation Officials (AASHTO), which provides guidance on roadway design,[22] and the *Manual on Uniform Traffic Control Devices,* which contains uniform standards for traffic control devices— date back as far as the late 1920s and 1930s. The primary focus was, and continues to be, on automobile and truck travel (Meyer and Dumbaugh 2004), although highway engineers are being encouraged by AASHTO and the Federal Highway Administration to interpret the guidelines more flexibly to better accommodate nonmotorized travel.

Design guidelines have evolved over the years, and many can accommodate the designs advocated for nonmotorized travel (Meyer and Dumbaugh 2004). The primary barrier appears to lie in how the standards have been implemented. The methods used to evaluate facility design requirements and performance, which are described in the following paragraphs, often tend to emphasize the needs of motorized travel at the expense of other modes (Meyer and Dumbaugh 2004).

---

[22] The Green Book is entitled *A Policy on Geometric Design of Highways and Streets* (AASHTO 2001).

Roadway design starts with a functional classification of highways into two environments—urban and rural—with three classes of roads under each—local roads, collectors, and arterials (AASHTO 2001).[23] Embedded in this framework are the competing concepts of access—the ability to travel to and from properties located adjacent to the travel way—and mobility—the ability to travel with a reasonable level of performance (i.e., at uncongested and reliable speeds) (Meyer and Dumbaugh 2004). Both of these concepts are oriented to vehicular travel with little attention to the nonmotorized traveler, who typically travels at low speeds for short distances.

Once a road has been classified, the design speed, or the speed at which motorized vehicles can travel safely on the road, is prescribed (Meyer and Dumbaugh 2004). The design speed then determines the other geometric elements of the road, such as its curvature. With the exception of local streets, the AASHTO Green Book exhorts the engineer to "use as high a design speed as practical" (AASHTO 2001, 67). Thus, many features compatible with pedestrian and bicycle travel, such as lower vehicle speeds and trees adjacent to the travel way, are viewed as limiting vehicular throughput and creating potentially dangerous obstacles should a vehicle leave the road, particularly on higher-speed roads (Meyer and Dumbaugh 2004).

Another decision involved in road design is determination of the "design vehicle," or the vehicle type that requires the greatest amount of maneuverability on a road. For example, if buses or trucks are expected to use a road, lane widths, turning radii, traffic signal timing, and the like will be oriented to these vehicle types. The resulting design facilitates higher operating and turning speeds for smaller passenger vehicles, which escalate the danger for pedestrians and cyclists who share the roads, and increases street-crossing distances for pedestrians and bicyclists (Meyer and Dumbaugh 2004).

---

[23] Local roads provide access to land with little or no through movement. Collectors collect traffic from local roads and connect them with higher-speed arterials. Arterials provide the highest level of service at the greatest speed for the longest uninterrupted distance, with some degree of access control (AASHTO 2001).

The demands placed on municipal street design to accommodate emergency vehicles and the implications for walking and cycling have already been discussed.

Vehicle-oriented performance measures affect both facility design and planned improvements. The level of service (LOS) is used to describe how a transportation facility is performing. It ranges from LOS A, defined as free flow where traffic volumes are low and there is little or no restriction on traffic flow, to LOS F, characterized as highly congested with stop-and-go traffic (AASHTO 2001). A desired LOS is used as a performance criterion in designing a facility and is then incorporated into development site guidelines, local comprehensive plans, and state policies. Existing roads that perform at or below the desired LOS are candidates for capacity enhancements whose primary objective is improved vehicular performance.

It is difficult to change both the vehicular orientation of road design and performance evaluation that favors higher ranges of design standards, which are equated with "better" and "safer" performance, and standardized approaches perceived by engineers as reducing liability claims (Meyer and Dumbaugh 2004). Nevertheless, AASHTO and the Federal Highway Administration have encouraged engineers to take advantage of existing guidelines by designing more flexibly to accommodate such objectives as nonmotorized travel on certain types of roads (see Meyer and Dumbaugh 2004 for further detail). Targeted approaches, such as context-sensitive design[24] and special design districts, make it possible to design roads to accommodate adjacent land uses and incorporate nonmotorized users for specific areas and projects without changing the entire underlying system of road classification and design criteria (see Box 4-6 for examples). Care must be taken to implement such projects with the safety of all users—motorized and nonmotorized—in mind so as not to increase the risk of crashes.

---

[24] Context-sensitive design is a project development process, including geometric design, that attempts to address safety and efficiency while being responsive to or consistent with a road's natural and human environment.

BOX 4-6

Two Examples of More Flexible
Transportation Infrastructure Design Approaches

Context-sensitive design. Many state transportation departments are moving toward a more flexible project design process known as context-sensitive design or, more broadly, context-sensitive solutions. This movement began in the late 1990s, when several states launched initiatives to define better ways of designing roadways. Perhaps one of the best definitions of context-sensitive design is found in a technical memorandum from the Minnesota Department of Transportation: "Context sensitive design is the art of creating public works that are well accepted by both the users and the neighboring communities. It integrates projects into the context or setting in a sensitive manner through careful planning, consideration of different perspectives and tailoring designs to particular project circumstances" (Minnesota Department of Transportation 2000). Such efforts are beginning to focus attention on those aspects of infrastructure design in sensitive community contexts that enable greater flexibility in implementing design standards.

Special design districts. Rather than relying on the ability of design professionals to arrive at the desired design ranges, some areas have attempted to circumvent the standardized roadway classification system through the creation of special design districts that indicate the desired dimensions for specific roads. Portland, Oregon, known for its progressive pedestrian orientation, included pedestrian districts as part of its original 1977 Arterial Streets Policy. These districts include special design criteria specifically addressing pedestrian travel (City of Portland 1998).

SOURCE: Meyer and Dumbaugh 2004.

Another common approach to accommodating nonmotorized travel is traffic calming. Originating in Europe, these measures are designed to slow traffic speeds in residential neighborhoods and near schools and pedestrian ways through self-enforcing physical devices. Examples are vertical deflections (speed humps and bumps and raised intersections); horizontal deflections (serpentines, bends, and deviations in a road); road narrowing (via neckdowns and chokers); and medians, central islands, and traffic circles (Loukaitou-Sideris 2004). The Institute of Transportation Engineers has developed suggested design guidelines for traffic calming measures encompassing applications, design and installation issues, potential impacts, and typical costs (ITE 2004).

Finally, more creative use of the cul-de-sac could be considered. Cul-de-sac patterns providing greater connectivity could achieve more of the benefits of the street grid pattern while retaining the cul-de-sac's higher levels of privacy, safety, and quiet and lower construction costs (Southworth and Ben-Joseph 2004). For example, designing residential communities that connected cul-de-sacs and loop streets through a system of pedestrian and bicycle paths would provide better access to parks, schools, and neighborhood shops (Southworth and Ben-Joseph 2004). Retrofitting existing suburban cul-de-sac developments could prove more difficult,[25] but "safe pathways" could be designed by using a combination of existing public rights-of-way, sidewalks, and street space in some closer-in suburbs.[26]

Transportation Infrastructure Financing

Transportation infrastructure financing has been a major factor in the development of the current transportation system. In particu-

---

[25] Building a pathway system to connect cul-de-sacs in a low-density suburban development would probably require building on private rights-of-way along lot lines. Single-use development limits the variety of destinations, although such paths could be used for exercise (Southworth and Ben-Joseph 2004).

[26] Locating community facilities and services on secondary streets should also improve traffic access for walking and cycling. Care must be exercised, however, not to congest residential areas or create a safety hazard for pedestrians and bicyclists.

lar, funding restrictions on use, matching shares, procedural requirements, and design standards all have had important influences on project outcomes. In general, nonmotorized transportation modes and, to a lesser extent, transit have not fared well in traditional programs and policies (Meyer and Dumbaugh 2004).

Funding arrangements differ across transportation modes. Highways have a well-established financing system with a long history of federal assistance, primarily from gas tax revenues set aside in the Highway Trust Fund. Local street and county road improvements, however, are financed from local revenues. Transit funding is a federal and local, and increasingly a state, responsibility. Nonmotorized transportation modes are primarily locally financed.

Different funding arrangements provide different incentives and constraints. For example, for many years the emphasis of federal-aid transportation programs was on highways, and matching requirements for state and local funds mirrored this emphasis. Federal funds financed 90 percent of Interstate highway construction, but only 50 to 80 percent of the cost of constructing transit facilities. In addition, projects using federal funds had to incorporate federally required design criteria. For many projects, this meant building an improved facility—adding more capacity for vehicular travel, for example—rather than simply replacing the existing facility as it was.

State and local funding arrangements vary widely by jurisdiction. For example, state constitutions restrict the majority of state gas tax revenues to highway expenditures. These projects rarely include pedestrian-oriented improvements, such as sidewalks, which are considered the responsibility of local governments or individual landowners (Meyer and Dumbaugh 2004).

Local governments have assumed many responsibilities for transportation financing, including nonmotorized modes. For example, many larger communities finance transit operations with sales tax set-asides approved by voter referendum. Bicycle paths and pedestrian facilities (e.g., street overpasses) are largely a local responsibility or the responsibility of individual landowners (e.g., sidewalks). Local governments can finance such improvements through local taxes or impact fees on new developments but are often reluctant to do so because of political backlash. These strategies shift costs directly to local residents (Meyer and Dumbaugh 2004).[27]

Since passage of the Intermodal Surface Transportation Efficiency Act of 1991 (ISTEA), the playing field between highways and transit has been leveled significantly. Certain highway funds can be "flexed" for transit and other nonhighway uses, and project matching shares for transit and highways are the same. In addition, several new programs were created that can help finance pedestrian and bicycle projects. One of the principal new funding sources for nonmotorized transportation is the Transportation Enhancements Program, which restricts 10 percent of Surface Transportation Program funds allocated to the states to such improvements as pedestrian and bicycle facilities and roadway beautification (Meyer and Dumbaugh 2004). The Congestion Mitigation and Air Quality Improvement (CMAQ) Program, also created by ISTEA, is aimed at improving metropolitan air quality. Projects such as bicycle, pedestrian, and transit improvements that encourage shifts from single-vehicle travel, thereby reducing vehicle emissions, are eligible for CMAQ funding (Meyer and Dumbaugh 2004). Another source of funding, particularly for enhancing bicycle and pedestrian safety, is the 402 program administered by the National Highway Traffic Safety Administration. Because sidewalks, intersection markings, and bicycle facilities can all be used to improve transportation safety, such projects are eligible for 402 funding (Meyer and Dumbaugh 2004). Finally, opportunities exist to incorporate pedestrian facilities and bicycle paths as part of other projects eligible for federal funding at minor additional cost.

REFERENCES

Abbreviations

AASHTO   American Association of State Highway and Transportation Officials
BR&S   Belden, Russonello & Stewart

---

[27] Developers typically build local streets and parking in subdivisions and charge back the home-owner-users. In the case of parking, this precludes shared parking and charging.

BTS   Bureau of Transportation Statistics
EPA   U.S. Environmental Protection Agency
FHA   Federal Housing Administration
DOT   U.S. Department of Transportation
ITE   Institute of Transportation Engineers
NRC   National Research Council
TRB   Transportation Research Board

AASHTO. 2001. *A Policy on Geometric Design of Highways and Streets,* 4th ed. Washington, D.C., Jan.

America Bikes. 2003. *Polls Show Americans Want Better Biking.* News release. Washington, D.C., May 5.

Appleyard, D. 1981. *Livable Streets.* University of California Press, Berkeley.

Barnes, P. M., and C. A. Schoenborn. 2003. Physical Activity Among Adults: United States, 2000. *Advance Data from Vital and Health Statistics,* No. 333, May 14.

Boarnet, M. G. 2004. *The Built Environment and Physical Activity: Empirical Methods and Data Resources.* Prepared for the Committee on Physical Activity, Health, Transportation, and Land Use, July 18.

Boarnet, M. G., and R. Crane. 2001. *Travel by Design: The Influence of Urban Form on Travel.* Oxford University Press, Inc., New York.

Boarnet, M. G., K. Day, C. Anderson, T. McMillen, and M. Alfonzo. 2004. Urban Form and Physical Activity: Insights from a Quasi-Experiment. Presented at the Active Living Research Annual Conference, Del Mar, Calif., Jan. 30.

Booth, M. L., N. Owen, A. Bauman, O. Clavis, and E. Leslie. 2000. Social-Cognitive and Perceived Environment Influences Associated with Physical Activity in Older Australians. *Preventive Medicine,* Vol. 31, No. 1, pp. 15–22.

Brown, J. D. 1992. Benefit Segmentation of the Fitness Market. Review. *Health Marketing Quarterly,* Vol. 9, No. 3–4, pp. 19–28.

Brownson, R. C., and T. K. Boehmer. 2004. *Patterns and Trends in Physical Activity, Occupation, Transportation, Land Use, and Sedentary Behaviors.* Department of Community Health and Prevention Research Center, School of Public Health, St. Louis University. Prepared for the Committee on Physical Activity, Health, Transportation, and Land Use, June 25.

Brownson, R. C., R. A. Housemann, D. R. Brown, J. Jackson-Thompson, A. C. King, B. R. Malone, and J. F. Sallis. 2000. Promoting Physical Activity in Rural Communities: Walking Trail Access, Use, and Effects. *American Journal of Preventive Medicine,* Vol. 18, pp. 235–241.

BR&S. 2003. *Americans' Attitudes Toward Walking and Creating Better Walking Communities.* Washington, D.C., April.

BTS. 2002. Bicycle Use Among Adult U.S. Residents. *OmniStats,* Vol. 2, Issue 6, U.S. Department of Transportation, Dec.

BTS. 2003. Pedestrian Travel During 2002. *OmniStats,* Vol. 3, Issue 1, U.S. Department of Transportation, July.

Calthorpe, P. 1993. *The Next American Metropolis: Ecology, Community, and the American Dream.* Princeton Architectural Press, New York.

City of Portland. 1998. *Portland Pedestrian Master Plan.* Office of Transportation, Engineering, and Development.

Collette, M., G. Godin, R. Bradet, and N. J. Gionet. 1994. Active Living in Communities: Understanding the Intention to Take Up Physical Activity as an Everyday Way of Life. *Canadian Journal of Public Health,* Vol. 85, No. 6, pp. 418–421.

Dellinger, A. M., and C. E. Staunton. 2002. Barriers to Children Walking and Cycling to School—United States, 1999. *Morbidity and Mortality Weekly Report,* Vol. 51, No. 32, Aug. 16, pp. 701–704.

DOT. 2003. *National Survey of Pedestrian and Bicyclist Attitudes and Behaviors—Highlights Report.* National Highway Traffic Safety Administration and Bureau of Transportation Statistics.

Duany, A., E. Plater-Zyberk, and J. Speck. 2000. *Suburban Nation: The Rise of Sprawl and the Decline of the American Dream.* North Point Press, N.J.

Dunn, A. L., B. H. Marcus, J. B. Kampert, M. E. Garcia, H. W. Kohl III, and S. N. Blair. 1999. Comparison of Lifestyle and Structured Interventions to Increase Physical Activity and Cardiorespiratory Fitness: A Randomized Trial. *Journal of the American Medical Association,* Vol. 281, pp. 327–334.

EPA. 2003. *Travel and Environmental Implications of School Siting.* EPA-231-R-03-004. Washington, D.C.

Eppli, M. J., and C. C. Tu. 1999. *Valuing the New Urbanism.* Urban Land Institute, Washington, D.C.

FHA. 1935. *Subdivision Development.* Circular No. 5, Washington, D.C., Jan. 10.

Fischel, W. A. 1999. Does the American Way of Zoning Cause the Suburbs of Metropolitan Areas to Be Too Spread Out? In *Governance and Opportunity in Metropolitan America* (A. Altshuler, W. Morrill, H. Wolman, and F. Mitchell, eds.), National Academy Press, Washington, D.C., pp. 151–191.

Fridinger, F., S. Kirby, E. Howze, W. Holmes, B. Latham, and B. Leonard. 1996. Nutrition and Physical Activity Communications at the Centers for Disease Control and Prevention. *Social Marketing Quarterly,* Vol. 3, No. 2, pp. 14–15.

Hahn, A., and E. Craythorn. 1994. Inactivity and the Physical Environment in Two Regional Centers. *Health Promotion Journal of Australia,* Vol. 4, No. 2, pp. 43–45.

Handy, S. 2004. *Critical Assessment of the Literature on the Relationships Among Transportation, Land Use, and Physical Activity*. Department of Environmental Science and Policy, University of California, Davis. Prepared for the Committee on Physical Activity, Health, Transportation, and Land Use, July.

Handy, S., M. G. Boarnet, R. Ewing, and R. E. Killingsworth. 2002. How the Built Environment Affects Physical Activity: Views from Urban Planning. *American Journal of Preventive Medicine*, Vol. 23, No. 2S, pp. 65–73.

ITE. 2004. Traffic Calming for Communities. www.ite.org/traffic. Accessed June 1, 2004.

Jackson, K. T. 1985. *Crabgrass Frontier: The Suburbanization of the United States*. Oxford University Press.

Jacobs, J. 1961. *The Death and Life of Great American Cities*. Random House, New York.

Jurgensmeyer, J., and T. Roberts. 1998. *Land Use Planning and Control Law*. West Group, St. Paul, Minn.

King, A. C., J. F. Sallis, A. L. Dunn, D. G. Simons-Morton, C. A. Albright, S. Cohen, W. J. Rejeski, B. H. Marcus, and M. C. Coday. 1998. Overview of the Activity Counseling Trial (ACT) Intervention for Promoting Physical Activity in Primary Health Care Settings. *Medicine and Science in Sports and Exercise*, Vol. 30, pp. 1086–1096.

King, A. C., C. Castro, S. Wilcox, A. A. Eyler, J. F. Sallis, and R. C. Brownson. 2000. Personal and Environmental Factors Associated with Physical Inactivity Among Different Racial Ethnic Groups of U.S. Middle-Aged and Older-Aged Women. *Health Psychology*, Vol. 19, No. 4, pp. 354–364.

Kirby, S. D., and M. Hollander. 2004. *Consumer Preferences and Social Marketing Approaches to Physical Activity Behavior and Transportation and Land Use Choices*. Prepared for the Committee on Physical Activity, Health, Transportation, and Land Use, April 20.

Kohl, H. W. III., A. L. Dunn, B. H. Marcus, and S. N. Blair. 1998. A Randomized Trial of Physical Activity Interventions: Design and Baseline Data from Project Active. *Medicine and Science in Sports and Exercise*, Vol. 30, pp. 275–283.

Kotler, P., N. Roberto, and N. Lee. 2002. Selecting Target Markets. In *Social Marketing: Improving the Quality of Life*, Sage Publications, Thousand Oaks, Calif., pp. 112–115.

Levine, J., and A. Inam. 2004. The Market for Transportation–Land Use Integration: Do Developers Want Smarter Growth Than Regulations Allow? *Transportation*, Vol. 31, pp. 409–427.

Logan, G. T., L. Frank, T. M. Noell, C. Leersen, and P. Engelke. 2001. *Overcoming Barriers to Smart Growth: Local Government Outreach Summary*. www.smartraq.net/pdfs/public%20officials.pdf.

Loukaitou-Sideris, A. 2004. *Transportation, Land Use, and Physical Activity: Safety and Security Considerations*. Prepared for the Committee on Physical Activity, Health, Transportation, and Land Use, June.

Meyer, M. D., and E. Dumbaugh. 2004. *Institutional and Regulatory Factors Related to Nonmotorized Travel and Walkable Communities.* Prepared for the Committee on Physical Activity, Health, Transportation, and Land Use, July.

Minnesota Department of Transportation. 2000. *Design Policy—Design Excellence Through Context Sensitive Design.* Technical Memorandum 00-24-TS-03. St. Paul.

NRC. 1999. *Governance and Opportunity in Metropolitan America* (A. Altshuler, W. Morrill, H. Wolman, and F. Mitchell, eds.), National Academy Press, Washington, D.C.

Portland Metro. 2000. *Light Rail Transit Station Zone.* Chapter 33. 450, Title 33, Oregon.

Pucher, J., and J. L. Renne. 2003. Socioeconomics of Urban Travel: Evidence from the 2001 NHTS. *Transportation Quarterly,* Vol. 57, No. 3, Summer, pp. 49–77.

Reger, B., L. Cooper, S. Booth-Butterfield, H. Smith, A. Bauman, M. Wootan, S. Middlestadt, B. Marcus, and F. Greet. 2002. WHEELING WALKS: A Community Campaign Using Paid Media to Encourage Walking Among Sedentary Older Adults. *Preventive Medicine,* Vol. 353, Sept., pp. 285–292.

Rudd, R. E., J. Goldberg, and W. Dietz. 1999. A Five-Stage Model for Sustaining a Community Campaign. *Journal of Health Communication,* Vol. 4, No. 1, pp. 37–48.

Schwanen, T., and P. Mokhtarian. 2004. What Affects Commute Mode Choice: Neighborhood Physical Structure or Preferences Toward Neighborhoods? *Journal of Transport Geography* (forthcoming).

Seneviratne, P. N. 1985. Acceptable Walking Distances in Central Areas. *Journal of Transportation Engineering,* Vol. 3, No. 4, pp. 365–376.

Shoup, D. 1994. Cashing Out Employer-Paid Parking: A Precedent for Congestion Pricing? In *Special Report 242: Curbing Gridlock: Peak-Period Fees to Relieve Traffic Congestion* (Vol. 2), National Research Council, Washington, D.C., pp. 152–199.

Shoup, D. 1997. Evaluating the Effects of Cashing Out Employer-Paid Parking: Eight Case Studies. *Transport Policy,* Vol. 4, No. 4, Oct., pp. 201–216.

Sloan, K. S. 2001. Physical Activity and 50+: Preliminary Findings to Support Effective Communications and Outreach. Presented at the Conference on Communicating Physical Activity and Health Messages: Science into Practice, Centers for Disease Control and Prevention and Health Canada, Dec. 8–11.

Smith-Heimer, J., and R. Golem. 2001. *Summary of Panel Discussions with California TOD Developers.* California Transit Authority, Statewide Transit-Oriented Development Study, Technical Appendix, pp. 128–139.

Southworth, M., and E. Ben-Joseph. 2004. Reconsidering the Cul-de-Sac. *Access,* No. 24, Spring, pp. 28–33.

Staunton, C., D. Hubsmith, and W. Kallins. 2003. Promoting Safe Walking and Biking to School. *American Journal of Public Health,* Vol. 93, No. 9, pp. 1431–1434.

TRB. 1994. *Special Report 242: Curbing Gridlock: Peak-Period Fees to Relieve Traffic Congestion.* National Research Council, Washington, D.C.

TRB. 1995. *Special Report 245: Expanding Metropolitan Highways: Implications for Air Quality and Energy Use.* National Research Council, Washington, D.C.

TRB. 2003. *Special Report 277: Measuring Personal Travel and Goods Movement: A Review of the Bureau of Transportation Statistics' Surveys.* National Research Council, Washington, D.C.

Wankel, L. M., and W. K. Mummery. 1993. Using National Survey Data Incorporating the Theory of Planned Behavior: Implications for Social Marketing Strategies in Physical Activity. *Journal of Applied Sport Psychology,* Vol. 5, No. 2, pp. 158–177.

Whyte, W. H. 1980. *The Social Life of Small Urban Spaces.* Conservation Foundation, Washington, D.C.

SUMMARY

Designing Research to Study the Relationship Between the Built Environment and Physical Activity

A more rigorous understanding of the extent to which the built environment is a factor in individuals' choices about physical activity is important in designing effective policies and interventions to address the decline in such activity. A review of the theory and data available to guide research on the links between the two reveals that conceptualization and measurement of the relevant environmental factors are a relatively new area of inquiry. A more complete theoretical framework is needed to provide the basis for formulating testable hypotheses, suggest the variables and relations for study, and help interpret study results.

Research designs emphasizing longitudinal approaches are particularly relevant for studying the potential causal relationship between a given aspect of the built environment and the desired behavior (i.e., more physical activity). With few exceptions, however, such studies are not evident in the research conducted to date. The issue of self-selection bias has only recently been incorporated into research designs. Both longitudinal and cross-sectional studies should use analytic approaches that help distinguish the extent to which an observed association between the built environment and physical activity reflects the characteristics of the built environment versus the attitudes and lifestyle preferences of those who choose to live in an environment with particular characteristics (e.g., walking and bicycle paths).

To date, most available research in this area has focused on cross-sectional analyses. The primary limitations of this research approach have been a poor understanding of the variables to include, which in turn reflects a deficiency of good theory, and the lack of well-developed measures of the relevant attributes of the built environment at the appropriate geographic scale. The latter can be traced to inadequate data, a function of the relatively immature stage of the research.

Measures of physical activity have been the focus of considerable research and are better developed than measures of the built environment. On the other hand, large surveys that measure physical activity and health have been focused primarily on leisure-time physical activity and do not provide information on the location of that activity. Thus, the researcher cannot determine total levels of physical activity or identify where the activity has occurred so these data can be linked with those on the characteristics of the built environment. At a minimum, geocoding the data collected in several of the large surveys on physical activity and health could facilitate linking these rich data sets with information on the built environment. Greater use of technologies that provide automated and objective measures to help verify the accuracy and enhance the precision of self-reported survey and diary data is already possible.

5

Designing Research to Study the Relationship Between the Built Environment and Physical Activity

As discussed in Chapter 4, the built environment can facilitate or constrain physical activity. This chapter is focused on designing research to provide a more rigorous understanding of how the built environment explains physical activity levels—the charge of this study. More important from a policy perspective, the discussion is concerned with issues of causality—the extent to which it can be said that the built environment affects physical activity, and the strength and magnitude of that effect. The chapter starts with an overview of the role of theory in studying the relationship between the built environment and physical activity. It then turns to a discussion of appropriate research designs and availability of data.[1]

THE ROLE OF THEORY

A theoretical framework that links the built environment to physical activity is critical to good research in this area. Theory provides the basis for formulating testable hypotheses and helps in the interpretation of results. It explains the subjects, variables, and relationships a researcher chooses to study.

---

[1] This chapter draws heavily on two papers commissioned for this study (Boarnet 2004 and Handy 2004). The reader is urged to consult these papers for more detailed exposition of many of the points raised in this chapter.

Indeed, one of the primary limitations of research to date on the relationship between the built environment and physical activity is the lack of an agreed-upon theoretical framework (Handy 2004). This deficiency is not surprising in view of the relatively recent interest in the topic and the fact that the necessary research must draw on expertise in at least two fields—public health and transportation. A recent review of the literature on the environmental factors associated with physical activity revealed that the conceptualization and measurement of environmental factors "comprise a relatively new area of research," and these attributes are "among the least understood of the known influences on physical activity" (Humpel et al. 2002, 188). The authors lay the problem squarely at the doorstep of inadequate theory: "Currently, even the most relevant theory does not provide sufficiently detailed conceptual tools for differentiating how the separate domains of environmental influences [e.g., accessibility, safety, aesthetics, weather] might impact on different physical activity behaviors" (Humpel et al. 2002, 197).

Research on travel behavior has drawn primarily on demand theory, as pioneered by McFadden (1974) in his Nobel prize–winning work on travel behavior modeling. The basic proposition, derived from economics and psychology, is that individuals make decisions in their self-interest, given the option to do so. In other words, most choices are made on the basis of their feasibility and their relative costs and benefits to the individual. Thus, for example, one would assume that people would be more likely to walk if walking trips became more pleasant, safer, or in any sense easier, or if alternatives to walking became more costly or more difficult.

This approach has been used primarily to forecast travel demand by motorized modes, generally for work trips and often at aggregate (regional) levels, to understand the likely impacts of alternative transportation investments on facility performance (Handy 2004). Demand theory is quite general in principle and can integrate individual perceptions and attitudes, detailed attributes of travel alternatives, and connections between short-term travel choices and long-term decisions about automobile ownership and residential and employment locations in consistent and counterintuitive ways. For example, the new-urbanist literature often states that denser neighborhoods will, intuitively, lead to less driving and more walking (e.g., Duany et al. 2000). Crane (1996a; 1996b), however, uses the demand framework to demonstrate that shorter trips actually stimulate trip taking by car, and the net result for both walking and driving is unclear. Yet walking and cycling have not been the focus of demand modeling to date, and hence the usefulness of the approach as a framework for understanding physical activity behavior has not been realized.

In summary, the main value of the demand approach is its power to explain how complex behaviors change with external circumstances. The way the utility-maximizing framework is commonly applied in modeling travel behavior would need to be altered for it to serve as an appropriate method for analyzing the relationship between the built environment and physical activity. Needed modifications include specifying benefits for walking and cycling as mode choices that are different from those for motorized travel. Minimizing travel time and cost and maximizing comfort are key determinants of motorized travel; the choice of walking or cycling depends more on the importance of combining exercise with utilitarian travel and minimizing the potential for collisions, temperature extremes, rainfall, and adverse terrain. In addition, characteristics of the built environment need to be incorporated into choice algorithms, as does day-to-day variation so that some minimum of walking or cycling time per week, for example, can be included in the overall travel pattern.

Health behavior research, including research on physical activity, has drawn heavily on theories from the field of psychology (Handy 2004). Social cognitive theory, developed by Bandura—an important influence on physical activity research—explains behavior as the interplay among the person, the behavior, and the environment in which the behavior is performed (Bandura 1986). Concepts such as the importance of perceptions and objective factors and the role of motivation and self-efficacy in overcoming barriers have been influential in understanding physical activity behavior. In general, the theory has emphasized the social rather than the physical environment (Handy 2004).

Ecological models evolved from social cognitive theory. The former emphasize the role of the physical as well as the social environment and thus extend social cognitive theory in ways that are more appropriate for analyzing the link between the built environment and physical activity (King et al. 2002; Sallis and Owen 2002). Ecological models, however, lack specificity about the characteristics of the built environment that might influence behavior. This lack of an agreed-upon conceptualization of the built environment helps explain the inconsistent approach to defining and measuring environmental variables in empirical research in this area, the subject of the next chapter.

Drawing heavily on both demand and ecological models, the committee developed its own conceptual model (see Figure 1-1 in Chapter 1). This scheme emphasizes a more detailed specification of both the built environment (e.g., different geographic scales, potentially relevant environmental characteristics at each scale) and physical activity (by type) (Figure 1-2). However, the specific elements of the model, such as the characteristics of the built environment, are illustrative rather than exhaustive.

RESEARCH DESIGNS

Appropriate research designs are also important in testing relationships among variables and in selecting relevant data. This section begins with a brief discussion of research design issues, particularly as they apply to the issue of establishing causal connections. Various research designs are then identified, their strengths and weaknesses are discussed, and their relevance in analyzing the link between the built environment and physical activity is considered.

Making the Causality Connection

The key question from a public health perspective is whether the built environment in place today affects physical activity in ways that are detrimental to health. As documented in Chapter 2, the causal link between adequate levels of physical activity and health is well established. The other half of the equation, the causal connection between the built environment and physical activity levels, is less well understood (Handy 2004; Boarnet 2004).

In considering research designs and evidence of causality in the relationship between the built environment and physical activity, there are several points to keep in mind. First, conclusions must be based on the results of many studies using a variety of research designs. All studies have weaknesses, and no single study will be sufficient to permit reaching conclusions. Second, the care with which research is performed is more important than the inherent strength or weakness of any given research design. A carefully conducted study with a weaker design generally is to be preferred over a less carefully conducted study with a better design. The care with which a study is performed is demonstrated in the theoretical underpinnings of the research, the use of the most appropriate design for the situation to be examined, the care with which exposures and outcomes are measured, consideration of biases, and the appropriateness of analytic methods.

Study Designs

By nature, causality is a time-ordered process: events or changes, such as an improvement in the built environment (e.g., the addition of a sidewalk), may have a consequence or effect (e.g., an increase in walking). Thus, time-series analyses generally provide the most appropriate research design for investigating cause-and-effect relationships.

Experimental Studies

The most persuasive scientific evidence of causality usually is derived from experimental studies of individuals. In such studies, subjects are randomly assigned to the exposures of interest and followed for the outcome of interest. The assignment to an exposure group is based on the needs of the study and not the participating individuals, although the risk of harm cannot knowingly be greater for members of any exposure group (Rothman and Greenland 1998). In the case of determining causal connections between the built environment and physical activity, the exposures would be to certain types of built environments, and the outcomes would be the types and amounts of physical activity performed. The important advantage of experimental studies is that researchers have considerable control over all aspects of the study, including the type of exposure, the selection of subjects, and the assignment of exposure to the subjects. When they are conducted well, experimental studies ensure that the exposure precedes the outcome, at least two doses of exposure are administered, and subjects are randomly assigned to exposure groups. This procedure minimizes the probability that the results and conclusions will be biased. Randomized clinical trials for drug testing are well-known examples of experimental studies.

Despite their advantages, experimental studies of individuals are not always possible. It is difficult to imagine, for example, how experimental studies of the relationship between the built environment and physical activity behaviors could be used to examine more than a small portion of the areas of interest. Modifying or creating new built environments just to conduct experimental research is, for practical purposes, impossible. Likewise, randomizing participants to specific residential or employment locations is implausible. Even if these barriers could be overcome, the limited, artificial, and intrusive nature of the experiment would likely jeopardize the generalizability of the results (Caporaso 1973). Similar limitations apply to laboratory experiments, which in this context could refer to asking subjects about their responses to hypothetical situations (e.g., preferences for different types of residential locations whose characteristics were systematically varied by the analyst's design)—referred to in the travel behavior literature as "stated preference" or "stated response" studies (Louviere et al. 2000). Fortunately, there are alternatives to experimental studies, commonly termed observational studies.

Observational Studies

Nonexperimental research designs are often referred to as observational studies because the researcher has little or no control over many aspects of the study and instead becomes a careful observer.

The terminology applied to the numerous designs of such studies varies across disciplines. A few of the most common designs and their main characteristics are reviewed here.

Longitudinal Studies Also called cohort, concurrent, follow-up, incidence, and prospective studies, longitudinal studies are those in which individuals have different levels of exposure to a variable of interest and are followed over time to determine the incidence of various outcomes. Two categories of longitudinal studies—quasi-experimental designs and natural experiments—deserve specific mention. Quasi-experimental designs are those in which the exposure is assigned but not according to a randomized experimental protocol. Investigators lack full control over the dose, timing, or allocation of subjects but conduct the study as if it were an experiment (Cook and Campbell 1979; Last et al. 2001). Natural experiments are situations in which differing groups in a population have differing exposures and can be observed for different outcomes (Last et al. 2001). Neither type of design is really an experiment because researchers have not randomly assigned the individuals to exposure groups. The terminology, while not strictly accurate, does call attention to the fact that human groups normally have different exposures and that these naturally occurring events can provide useful information.

An example of a natural experiment is discussed by Boarnet (2004). The California Safe Routes to School Program (see Box 4-1 in Chapter 4) awarded construction funds to numerous communities to improve the safety and viability of walking and cycling to school. A large number of projects (186) that involved changing the built environment were funded within a period of a few years (two annual award cycles). This created the opportunity for a natural-experimental research design. The results are reported in Chapter 4, but in his commissioned paper, Boarnet (2004) makes several suggestions concerning research design that are relevant to the present discussion. First, several projects should be studied because single projects may encounter practical difficulties (e.g., construction delays). In addition, studying an array of projects improves the ability to generalize the results. Second, before-and-after studies must have baseline data. Ideally, these data should be collected before the intervention occurs. An alternative, second-best approach is to ask subjects retrospectively to compare their activity levels before and after the improvement. Finally, natural experiments may involve groups that have different exposures, but in many such studies, this does not occur by design. For example, Boarnet (2004) found that most but not all of the construction projects he reviewed had been located in places where children would come into contact with them on the way to school. That distinction enabled the researchers to develop ad hoc intervention and nonintervention groups on the basis of whether the children would pass the project on their usual route to school.

Case-Control Studies In case-control studies, exposure to an acknowledged risk factor is compared between individuals from the same population with and without a condition. As opposed to longitudinal studies, in which participants are enrolled and grouped according to exposure status, in case-control studies participants are grouped according to their outcome status. This could mean, for example, sorting individuals on the basis of their activity level (e.g., active versus sedentary) into case and control groups to see whether there are statistically significant differences in environmental characteristics that may influence the propensity of the two groups to be physically active.

Cross-Sectional Studies Also called prevalence studies, cross-sectional studies examine the relationship between conditions (e.g., physical activity behaviors) and other variables of interest in a defined population at a single point in time. For example, the physical activity behavior of matched pairs of individuals and communities could be compared at a particular point in time. Thus the walking and cycling behavior of individuals in a more pedestrian-oriented neighborhood could be compared with that of individuals in a typical suburban planned unit development. The communities could be matched by income, location, accessibility to transportation services, and topography to isolate the characteristics associated with the friendliness of the different communities to walking and cycling and the potential effect of those characteristics on these activities. Such cross-sectional studies can quantify the presence and magnitude of associations between variables. Unlike longitudinal studies, however, they cannot be used to determine the temporal relationship between variables, and evidence of cause and effect cannot be assumed. As discussed in the following chapter, most studies of the built environment and physical activity have been cross-sectional.

Other Research Design Issues

Level of Aggregation and Geographic Scale

Aggregate data are rarely helpful in illuminating causal links. Because physical activity manifests itself at the individual level, one could argue that the individual is the proper unit of analysis. As shown in the committee's detailed conceptual model (Figure 1-2 in Chapter 1), physical activity is undertaken at many geographic scales—in and around the home, at work, in facilities such as schools and recreation centers, in the neighborhood, and in the region. This adds a layer of complexity.

As hypothesized in Figure 1-2, at each geographic scale different features of the built environment may have different effects on the individual's propensity to be physically active. Short distances providing easy access to multiple destinations and a pleasant and safe environment may be important facilitators of physical activity in the neighborhood. By comparison, the size and distribution of activities in a metropolitan area and the availability of transportation alternatives to the automobile (e.g., transit) may dominate the extent to which one chooses a physically active mode of transportation for regional travel, such as commuting or traveling to a shopping center.

Furthermore, the effect of the built environment is likely to differ by type of physical activity. Safety and access to parks and other recreational facilities, for example, may be important in encouraging leisure-time physical activity outside the home. On the other hand, time and distance are likely to be more important factors in the decision to use nonmotorized transport for destination-oriented travel and may also affect destination choice.

Because most physical activity is spatially constrained and bounded by peoples' time budgets and physical limitations, smaller geographic units of analysis (e.g., neighborhoods, areas around work sites) are likely to yield more information on the attributes of the built environment that influence physical activity. In general, as discussed in more detail in the next chapter, issues of geographic scale have been underexamined in recent studies linking physical activity behavior to the built environment (Boarnet 2004).

Self-Selection

A basic research challenge is distinguishing the role of personal attitudes, preferences, and motivations and of external influences in observed behavior. For example, do people walk more in a particular neighborhood because of pleasant tree-lined sidewalks, or do they live in a neighborhood with pleasant tree-lined sidewalks because they like to walk? This "self-selection" problem potentially confounds the ability of researchers to distinguish how much walking and cycling in an activity-friendly neighborhood is associated with the built environment and how much reflects the attitudes and lifestyle preferences of those who choose to live there. In his paper, Boarnet (2004, 4) raises this point specifically:

> Persons might choose their environments in part based on their desired level of physical activity. It does not take much imagination to believe that an avid surfer would choose to live near the beach or that a ski enthusiast would move near the mountains. Generalizing to other, more common forms of physical activity, do persons who wish to walk choose residences in pedestrian-oriented neighborhoods near parks? If so, the association between physical activity and urban form might represent persons' residential location choices rather than an influence of the built environment on activity.

If researchers do not properly account for the choice of neighborhood, their empirical results will be biased in the sense that features of the built environment may appear to influence activity more than they in fact do. (Indeed, this single potential source of statistical bias casts doubt on the majority of studies on the topic to date; see Chapter 6.) Various researchers have tried to control for the possibility of self-selection bias in a number of ways. Boarnet and Sarmiento (1998) and Boarnet and Crane (2001a; 2001b) used instrumental-variables techniques to control for choice of residential location in studying how neighborhood features shape motorized travel.[2] Bagley and Mokhtarian (2002) used structural-equations modeling[3] to account simultaneously for multiple directions of causality, such as the influence of attitudes on both travel and residential location, and the influence of residential location on travel behavior once attitudes were controlled for. Cervero and Duncan (2002) examined mode choice among residents of transit-oriented developments by using nested logit techniques. In their analysis, mode choice was expressed hierarchically as a function of residential location, which in turn was expressed as a function of workplace location.

Another strategy for coping with self-selection bias is to observe when a person moves and to draw associations between changes in the built environment near that person's new residence vis-à-vis the old and changes in physical activity levels. Krizek (2003) employed such an approach in studying influences of urban design on travel behavior. Research in progress by Handy and Mokhtarian is also focusing on the travel behavior of recent movers to a variety of types of neighborhoods compared with that of a similar group of non-movers in the same neighborhoods. However, moving is often associated with other life changes—marital status, job change, family size, and age of children—that can confound the effect of the new environment on changes in physical activity levels (Boarnet 2004).

---

[2] This technique involves regression analysis with multiple endogenous variables. In addition, the researcher must have some variables that influence housing location choice but do not also influence the decision to be physically active. Because many sociodemographic characteristics that influence residential location also influence an individual's choice to be physically active, care must be taken in specifying the regression models (Boarnet 2004).

[3] This approach involves estimating coefficients for multiple interrelated equations at a time, where each equation represents a hypothesized direction of causality. It can account for not only the direct effects of one variable on another but also indirect effects through intermediate variables.

Another approach is to focus on children under the assumption that children do not choose their residential location. An important consideration, however, is that parents may impart attitudes about physical activity to their children. For example, if parents prefer and choose to live in an activity-friendly location, correlations between the child's level of physical activity and the built environment may not demonstrate an independent causal effect, but rather reflect the parental attitudes that have been transmitted to the child (Boarnet 2004). Natural experiments, discussed earlier in this chapter, are another way of circumventing potential self-selection bias. The change in the built environment in such a study, however, cannot be so large as to induce residential relocation, thus confounding the independent effect of the change in the built environment on physical activity levels (Boarnet 2004).

Finally, Schwanen and Mokhtarian approached this issue in a series of studies by comparing the travel behavior of "matched" (or "consonant") residents of urban and suburban neighborhoods (that is, those who are living in the type of neighborhood they prefer) with that of "mismatched" or "dissonant" residents. They examined the question of whether the travel behavior of mismatched individuals is more like that of the matched residents of the neighborhood in which they actually live or that of the matched residents of the kind of neighborhood in which they would prefer to live. The former outcome would suggest that the effects of the built environment outweigh personal predispositions, while the latter would suggest the converse. Schwanen and Mokhtarian (2003) compared non-commute-trip frequencies of matched and mismatched urban and suburban residents, Schwanen and Mokhtarian (2004a) compared the commute mode choice of consonant and dissonant workers, and Schwanen and Mokhtarian (2004b) completed the picture by examining the role of dissonance in mode-specific distances traveled for all purposes.

Efforts to address the issue of self-selection specifically have only recently been incorporated into research on the influences of the built environment on physical activity. Thus, much remains to be learned about the issue's relative importance. (Economics and political science have a considerable literature on residential self-selection that could be drawn upon.[4]) Knowledge gained through a combination of analytical methods, whether econometric tools or natural experiments, should shed considerable light on this question. Until a body of evidence takes form and the importance of this issue is better understood, the ability to link features of the built environment to physical activity levels will necessarily remain limited.

Validity

Two other important hallmarks of good research design are internal and external validity. Internal validity is the degree to which the research design accurately and faithfully reflects the conceptual model that guides the empirical study. Most important, all necessary control variables are used to remove confounding influences and reduce the chances of spurious inferences. Data limitations rarely allow this to be done for a topic such as built environments and physical activity—an issue addressed in the following section. The validity of the data, which is also a concern, is discussed below.

External validity speaks to the generalizability of the research. Data drawn from a single case (e.g., one city or a particular neighborhood) have often been used in past empirical research on the link between the built environment and physical activity levels. As a substantial body of research drawn from many cities and settings accumulates, the external validity of research in this area should improve.

AVAILABILITY OF DATA

Lack of data is one of the main barriers to further progress in examining the causal links between the built environment and physical activity levels. Just as the development of an appropriate theoretical framework will require the joint involvement of the public health and transportation communities, so, too, will the development of appropriately linked data sets. The first grants from the Robert

---

[4] For example, Tiebout (1956) and others posit that residents self-select into jurisdictions offering packages of public services that match their preferences (NRC 1999).

Wood Johnson Foundation's Active Living Research Program were earmarked entirely for the development of reliable measures of both the built environment and physical activity, an illustration of the importance of data and measurement to research.[5]

Measurement Issues

Many measurement issues affect the ability of a researcher to measure the link between the built environment and physical activity (see also Chapter 2). The first such issue relates to the trade-off between the precision and accuracy of the data and their breadth and accessibility. For example, physical activity can be measured directly as energy expenditure by methods that gauge metabolic energy rates. Pedometers, which count steps and measure distance, and accelerometers, which measure the intensity of an activity, provide objective but somewhat less precise measures of physical activity than those obtained with metabolic methods.[6] Indirect measures of physical activity rely on self-reports from surveys or diaries. Of course, direct laboratory measures are the most precise, but they are also the most costly, inconvenient, and artificial (i.e., the results may not be representative of real-life contexts). Use of pedometers and accelerometers, particularly to supplement and corroborate survey data, is less demanding but risks a possible "Hawthorne effect": respondents must wear the devices and may change their activity patterns because they know they are being monitored.[7] Surveys are the most efficient way of collecting data

---

[5] Grants were available to (*a*) develop and evaluate objective measures of urban and suburban land use variables that are believed to be related to physical activity; (*b*) develop and evaluate objective measures of the physical characteristics of green spaces, parks, walking trails, and other public recreational areas and open spaces that may be associated with physical activity; (*c*) assess physical activity in specific environments, such as trails, sidewalks, and stairways; and (*d*) develop and validate combined measures of travel behavior and physical activity (RWJF 2002).

[6] Pedometers have been shown to provide a valid measure of distance walked, but they are not useful for measuring many other types of physical activity. Because they are typically worn at the hip, accelerometers provide more accurate measures of lower body movement, such as walking and running, than of upper body movement, such as shoveling or sweeping (Boarnet 2004).

[7] "Hawthorne effect" refers to the alteration of human behavior because subjects know they are being studied. This effect was first demonstrated in a research project of the Hawthorne Plant of Western Electric Company in Cicero, Illinois.

needed from large numbers of respondents in a range of environments if the objective is to examine the effect of the built environment on physical activity and health outcomes. However, the data collected from surveys and diaries are self-reported, so accuracy and bias are concerns. One commonly used technique to address the accuracy issue is to calibrate survey-collected measures of physical activity against laboratory measures (Boarnet 2004).

A second measurement issue relates to the need for objective as well as subjective measures. This distinction is more important for measures of the built environment than for measures of physical activity.[8] Geographic information systems (GIS) now widely available can provide objective measures of many features of the built environment, such as street connectivity and the presence and location of sidewalks, parks, open spaces, and schools (Boarnet 2004).[9] As discussed in the preceding chapter, however, individuals' perceptions of their environment are also important to their choices about being physically active. Thus data on subjective factors, such as individuals' perceptions of neighborhood safety and the quality of amenities that encourage them to walk and cycle, are an important complement to objective measures. Research is under way to develop more standardized protocols for measuring the perceived qualities of the built environment (see Winston et al. 2004, for example).

A third measurement issue relates to the scale of the data, in particular, the need for fine-grained data on features of the built environment because much physical activity is undertaken near one's home and workplace. GIS measures of the built environment have become common in studies of land use and travel behavior. They yield geographic-linked data on population and employment densities, mix of commercial and residential land uses, and characteristics of street networks (e.g., street grids, four-way intersections) (Boarnet 2004). However, just because objective data exist in a GIS for an area does not mean that the data are on appropriate variables

---

[8] People's perception of how active they are is less important than an objective measure of how active they really are.

[9] A geographic information system is an automated system for the capture, storage, retrieval, analysis, and display of spatial data.

or at scales that are useful for analyzing the relationship between the built environment and physical activity.

Two other measurement issues relate to the reliability and validity of the data. Reliability refers to the likelihood that a data measure or survey instrument will provide the same result when it is used by a different researcher or in a different test. For example, interrater reliability is frequently measured when the research involves environmental audits—direct observation of the built environment that is accomplished by walking neighborhoods and recording information about selected environmental characteristics. (See Box 5-1 for an example of an environmental audit instrument.) Va-

---

BOX 5-1

The Systematic Pedestrian and Cycling Environmental Scan Instrument

The Systematic Pedestrian and Cycling Environmental Scan Instrument, or SPACES, is one of the first environmental audit instruments developed to measure features of the built environment associated with physical activity (Pikora et al. 2002). To use the SPACES audit tool, observers walk through neighborhoods answering questions that prompt them to record information about street width, sidewalks, traffic volume, lighting, aesthetics, parks and shops, and various other factors that might be linked to physical activity. Information is recorded for individual blocks and thus can be aggregated to higher geographic levels or analyzed at the block level. The SPACES audit tool has been reliability tested, and Pikora et al. (2002) report that many of the questions have high interrater reliability.

A similar audit tool, also applied at the block level, was developed to measure the built environment near school sites in the evaluation of the California Safe Routes to School Program (see Box 4-1 in Chapter 4) (Boarnet et al. 2003).

SOURCE: Boarnet 2004.

lidity refers to an assessment of whether the data collected are accurate relative to some objective standard or measure. For example, as noted above, accelerometers are considered an objective measure of the intensity of physical activity, but their accuracy falls short when validated with portable metabolic units; accelerometers may underestimate energy expenditure by one-third to two-thirds of the more objective metabolic measurement (Welk 2002 in Boarnet 2004). Likewise, the validity of self-reported survey or diary data on travel and other forms of physical activity is problematic because subject recall may be faulty or biased or both. The Strategies for Metro Atlanta's Regional Transportation and Air Quality (SMARTRAQ) project is an example of an approach that supplements self-reported data on walking and other nonmotorized transport collected from travel diaries with the use of more objective Global Positioning System (GPS)[10] data and accelerometers as a check on the location and intensity of the physical activity (see Box 5-2).

The above measurement issues affect the quality of the data available to study the link between the built environment and physical activity. Another, more fundamental challenge is to link disparate databases and data on the built environment and physical activity for research purposes. Currently, these data are spread across a variety of data sources from different fields that have often been developed to address different questions (Boarnet 2004).

Data on Physical Activity

Despite the limitations noted above and in Chapter 2, surveys are the most promising sources of data for studying the links among the built environment, physical activity, and health (Boarnet 2004). The principal public health surveys, identified and discussed in Chapter 2, offer national-level data on a range of physical activity that are tracked over time and are readily available to researchers.[11]

---

[10] GPS is a worldwide radionavigation system comprising a constellation of 24 satellites and their ground stations. GPS uses these "man-made stars" as reference points to calculate positions accurate to the level of meters.

[11] These surveys do not track the same sample of individuals over time and thus should not be confused with true longitudinal studies.

BOX 5-2

Strategies for Metro Atlanta's Regional Transportation and Air Quality

SMARTRAQ was an attempt to link travel diary surveys with information on physical activity. Typically, travel diaries collect self-reported data on walking and cycling but have little objective data on these or other types of physical activity. Nor is specific information generally available about the location where the activity occurred.

As part of a comprehensive travel diary study, SMARTRAQ equipped 500 respondents with GPS transponders and accelerometers. The GPS units were shoulder-mounted systems that tracked walking and other nonmotorized travel. Accelerometers provided measures of activity that did not rely on self-reports. GPS provided information on location that allowed a detailed linking to the built environment, while the accelerometer gave information about the intensity of the physical activity. These two data sources offered the potential to yield information about the link between physical activity and the built environment while also providing a prototype for future studies. More information about SMARTRAQ is presented in the appendix of the paper by Boarnet (2004).

SOURCE: Boarnet 2004.

One limitation of these databases is incomplete coverage of physical activity. As noted in Chapter 2, the major focus of public health surveys has been on leisure-time physical activity. Only recently have data on utilitarian travel begun to be included, but these data are not recorded separately, and physical activity at the workplace is not reported at all. Another key gap, which reflects the early stage of interest in and research on the links among physical activity, health, and the built environment, is the lack of any reported geographic or environmental data that would enable researchers to link survey information on physical activity levels with details about the respondent's location and physical environment.

These limitations can be addressed. More comprehensive measures of physical activity are being collected in many public health surveys (see, for example, the discussion of the Behavioral Risk Factor Surveillance System in Chapter 2). Geocoding of physical activity and health survey data using GIS is probably the most efficient way to provide the needed links to data on the built environment (Boarnet 2004). Of course, issues of subject anonymity and confidentiality must be addressed, but there are precedents for doing so.

Data on the Built Environment and Travel

Data on the built environment are not as well developed as data on physical activity and health. Standardized data sets on the built environment are rare, even at the metropolitan area level (Boarnet 2004) (see Box 5-3 for two examples of local land use databases). Typically, researchers must construct such data sets by using available GIS data supplemented with observational environmental audits when necessary and feasible.

Testing of the accuracy of measures of the built environment is at a preliminary stage relative to measures of physical activity. In particular, as discussed in the next chapter, additional research is needed to determine which elements of the built environment are most useful for studying the environmental determinants of physical activity (Boarnet 2004). Complicating this task is the need for fine-grained measures of environmental features (e.g., size and orientation of parking lots, availability and condition of sidewalks), as well as of related mediating variables that may affect individual decisions to be physically active, such as local crime rates and the amount and speed of traffic (Boarnet 2004).

Data on land use and travel behavior are available but typically have not focused on the full range of physical activities and offer limited geographic detail. The National Household Transportation Survey—the primary source of data on nationwide travel behavior—covers commuting as well as nonwork travel, including

BOX 5-3

Examples of GIS-Based Land Use
and Built Environment Databases

One of the better examples of GIS-based land use databases is the Regional Land Information System (RLIS) for metropolitan Portland, Oregon. The Portland Metro has been developing this sophisticated GIS land use database for more than 10 years. The RLIS database includes GIS-based data on sidewalks, bicycle routes, rivers, paths, vegetation cover, slopes, parks, and open spaces, linked to both street and census geography. This is an advanced set of geographic data that enables researchers to use measures of the built and natural environments without having to develop those measures on their own. (See Bolen 2002 for more detail on RLIS.)

Montgomery County, Maryland, is also a leader in making advanced GIS-based land use data available to the research community. The county has developed a website that provides land use information and, in many cases, GIS-compatible land use data. These data include parcel-level information on land uses, aerial photographs that can illustrate detailed historical land use patterns, street maps, bicycle paths, parks, ball fields, watersheds and other natural resources, open spaces, job access, and school boundaries.

The experience in Portland and Montgomery County suggests that evolving best practices for metropolitan land use data will include the following: parcel-level land use and zoning data supplemented with aerial photographs and remote sensing data; land use information for individual parcels that allows the calculation of land use mix; street networks; sidewalk coverage; bicycle paths; parks and other recreation areas; natural resources such as waterways, lakes, and open spaces; accessibility measures that include access to jobs and shopping; school boundaries; crime rates; street lighting; and street tree coverage and other features that provide shelter from the elements. As communities digitize existing databases, such detailed information will become increasingly common. Best practices in GIS-based land use and built environment databases will include user-friendly website access and download capability, data that are compatible with common GIS programs, and historical land use and built environment data that enable changes to be tracked.

SOURCE: Boarnet 2004.

walking and cycling. As discussed in Chapter 2, the 2001 survey attempted to get a better handle on walking, the most common form of physical activity. Plans are to release block-level and census tract data to researchers in 2004, pending completion of confidentiality agreements and the availability of funding to support the data release (Boarnet 2004). Thus for the first time in the United States, researchers will be able to study the relationship between travel and the built environment at the neighborhood level.

At the local level, many metropolitan planning organizations (MPOs) conduct periodic travel diary surveys to provide input into the development and updating of regional travel forecasting models. Typically, the larger MPOs have geocoded the data so a researcher can link them to data on the built environment. Geographically based information about the survey respondent— either residential location or the locations of trip origins and destinations—can be linked to census data on socioeconomic characteristics or to other information about the built environment.[12] Use of travel diaries is limited by the fact that most diary surveys collect self-reported data on walking and cycling but few data on other types of physical activity (e.g., gardening, housework, stair climbing) (Boarnet 2004). The SMARTRAQ project, described in Box 5-2, is a promising exception.

Linking Data on the Built Environment and Physical Activity

Modifying existing national survey data on physical activity and health so they can be linked geographically to measures of the built environment is the most immediate improvement likely to provide researchers with the necessary data to better understand potential causal links between physical activity and urban form (Boarnet 2004). Refining measures of both physical activity and the built environment is another important step (Boarnet 2004). Measures of the former are more advanced, but completeness is an issue if total physical activity levels are to be studied. Greater attention should

---

[12] See Handy and Clifton (2001) and Greenwald and Boarnet (2001) for examples of the use of these techniques.

be focused on capturing physical activity for utilitarian purposes as well as for recreation and exercise, and both types of data should encompass activities in and around the home and workplace, which currently are understudied areas. Devising appropriate and valid measures of the built environment—in particular, developing a better understanding of which features are likely to influence physical activity levels—is a greater challenge. Fine-grained measures of features of the built environment that support physical activity—pedestrian and bicycle paths, public spaces, street lighting at both the neighborhood and workplace levels—may not be available in GIS maps in some localities and may require additional data collection (Boarnet 2004).[13] Once more standardized measures are developed, it should be easier to test hypotheses about the relative effect of various characteristics of the built environment on physical activity levels in a range of settings.

REFERENCES

Abbreviations

NRC   National Research Council
RWJF   Robert Wood Johnson Foundation

Bagley, M. N., and P. L. Mokhtarian. 2002. The Impact of Neighborhood Type on Travel Behavior: A Structural Equations Modeling Approach. *Annals of Regional Science,* Vol. 36, No. 2, pp. 279–297.

Bandura, A. 1986. *Social Foundations of Thought and Action: A Social Cognitive Theory.* Prentice-Hall, Inc., Englewood Cliffs, N.J.

Boarnet, M. G. 2004. *The Built Environment and Physical Activity: Empirical Methods and Data Resources.* Prepared for the Committee on Physical Activity, Health, Transportation, and Land Use, July 18.

Boarnet, M. G., and R. Crane. 2001a. The Influence of Urban Form on Travel: Specification and Estimation Issues. *Transportation Research A,* Vol. 35, No. 9, pp. 823–845.

Boarnet, M. G., and R. Crane. 2001b. *Travel by Design: The Influence of Urban Form on Travel.* Oxford University Press, Inc., New York.

---

[13] Two options for collecting these additional data are the use of remote sensing or aerial photography and direct observation through an environmental audit (Boarnet 2004).

Boarnet, M. G., K. Day, C. Anderson, T. McMillan, and M. Alfonzo. 2003. *Safe Routes to School*, Vols. 1 and 2. California Department of Transportation, Sacramento, Dec.

Boarnet, M. G., and S. Sarmiento. 1998. Can Land Use Policy Really Affect Travel Behavior? A Study of the Link Between Non-Work Travel and Land Use Characteristics. *Urban Studies*, Vol. 35, No. 7, pp. 1155–1169.

Bolen, R. 2002. *GIS: Essential for Urban Growth Management: Portland, Oregon Metropolitan Area*. Presented at RLIS@Ten Symposium, Portland, Ore., March. www.metro-region.org/library_docs/maps_data/gis_and_planning.pdf. Accessed Nov. 18, 2003.

Caporaso, J. A. 1973. Quasi-Experimental Approaches to Social Science: Perspectives and Problems. In *Quasi-Experimental Approaches: Testing Theory and Evaluating Policy* (J. A. Caporaso and L. L. Roos, Jr., eds.), Northwestern University Press, Evanston, Ill., Chapter 1.

Cervero, R., and M. Duncan. 2002. *Residential Self Selection and Rail Commuting: A Nested Logit Analysis*. University of California Working Paper. www.uctc.net/papers/604.pdf.

Cook, T. D., and O. T. Campbell. 1979. *Quasi-Experimentation*. Rand McNally, Chicago.

Crane, R. 1996a. Cars and Drivers in the New Suburbs. *Journal of the American Planning Association*, Vol. 62, pp. 51–65.

Crane, R. 1996b. On Form Versus Function: Will the New Urbanism Reduce Traffic, or Increase It? *Journal of Planning Education and Research*, Vol. 15, pp. 117–126.

Duany, A., E. Plater-Zyberk, and J. Speck. 2000. *Suburban Nation: The Rise of Sprawl and the Decline of the American Dream*. North Point Press, N.J.

Greenwald, M. J., and M. G. Boarnet. 2001. Built Environment as Determinant of Walking Behavior: Analyzing Nonwork Pedestrian Travel in Portland, Oregon. In *Transportation Research Record: Journal of the Transportation Research Board, No. 1780*, TRB, National Research Council, Washington, D.C., pp. 33–42.

Handy, S. 2004. *Critical Assessment of the Literature on the Relationships Among Transportation, Land Use, and Physical Activity*. Prepared for the Committee on Physical Activity, Health, Transportation, and Land Use, July.

Handy, S., and K. Clifton. 2001. Local Shopping as a Strategy for Reducing Automobile Travel. *Transportation*, Vol. 28, No. 4, pp. 317–346.

Humpel, N., N. Owen, and E. Leslie. 2002. Environmental Factors Associated with Adults' Participation in Physical Activity. *American Journal of Preventive Medicine*, Vol. 22, No. 3, pp. 188–199.

King, A. C., D. Stokols, E. Talen, G. S. Brassington, and R. Killingsworth. 2002. Theoretical Approaches to the Promotion of Physical Activity: Forging a Transdisciplinary Paradigm. *American Journal of Preventive Medicine*, Vol. 23, No. 2S, pp. 15–25.

Krizek, K. 2003. Residential Relocation and Changes in Urban Travel: Does Neighborhood-Scale Urban Form Matter? *Journal of the American Planning Association*, Vol. 69, No. 3, pp. 265–281.

Last, J. M., R. A. Spasoff, S. S. Harris, and M. C. Thuriaux. 2001. *A Dictionary of Epidemiology,* 4th ed. Oxford University Press.

Louviere, J. J., D. A. Hensher, and J. D. Swait. 2000. *Stated Choice Methods: Analysis and Application.* Cambridge University Press, Cambridge, United Kingdom.

McFadden, D. L. 1974. The Measurement of Urban Travel Demand. *Journal of Public Economics,* Vol. 3, pp. 303–328.

NRC. 1999. *Governance and Opportunity in Metropolitan America* (A. Altshuler, W. Morrill, H. Wolman, and F. Mitchell, eds.), National Academy Press, Washington, D.C.

Pikora, T. J., F. C. L. Bull, K. Jamrozik, M. Knuiman, B. Giles-Corti, and R. J. Donovan. 2002. Developing a Reliable Audit Instrument to Measure the Physical Environment for Physical Activity. *American Journal of Preventive Medicine,* Vol. 23, No. 3, pp. 187–194.

Rothman, K. J., and S. Greenland. 1998. *Modern Epidemiology.* Lippincott-Raven, Philadelphia, Pa.

RWJF. 2002. *Active Living Policy and Environmental Studies Program Special Solicitation.* Princeton, N.J., May.

Sallis, J. F., and N. Owen. 2002. Ecological Models of Health Behavior. In *Health Behavior and Health Education: Theory, Research, and Practice* (K. Glanz, B. K. Rimer, and F. M. Lewis, eds.), Jossey-Bass, San Francisco, Calif.

Schwanen, T., and P. L. Mokhtarian. 2003. Does Dissonance Between Desired and Current Neighborhood Type Affect Individual Travel Behavior? An Empirical Assessment from the San Francisco Bay Area. *Proceedings of the European Transport Conference,* Strasbourg, France, Oct. 8–10. www.its.ucdavis.edu/publications/2003/RP-03-18.pdf.

Schwanen, T., and P. L. Mokhtarian. 2004a. What Affects Commute Mode Choice: Neighborhood Physical Structure or Preferences Toward Neighborhoods? *Journal of Transport Geography,* forthcoming.

Schwanen, T., and P. L. Mokhtarian. 2004b. What If You Live in the Wrong Neighborhood? The Impact of Residential Neighborhood Type Dissonance on Distance Traveled. Submitted for publication.

Tiebout, C. 1956. A Pure Theory of Local Expenditures. *Journal of Political Economy,* Vol. 64, Oct., pp. 416–424.

Welk, G. J. 2002. Use of Accelerometry-Based Activity Monitors to Assess Physical Activity. In *Physical Activity Assessments for Health-Related Research* (G. J. Welk, ed.), Human Kinetics, Champaign, Ill.

Winston, E., R. Ewing, and S. Handy. 2004. The Built Environment and Active Travel: Developing Measures of Perceptual Urban Design Qualities. Presented at 83rd Annual Meeting of the Transportation Research Board, Washington, D.C.

SUMMARY

Current State of Knowledge

A review of the empirical evidence on the relationship between the built environment and physical activity levels indicates this to be a relatively new field of inquiry. The work conducted to date has embodied two strands of research—one from urban planning and travel behavior and the other from public health and physical activity. Addressing the topic from a broad range of perspectives, areas of expertise, and measures of the variables of interest has stimulated the contributions of a wide range of researchers. In the absence of a common conceptual framework, a more standardized vocabulary, and better linked data sets, however (see Chapter 5), the majority of studies remain at the correlates stage.

The literature provides a growing body of evidence that shows an association between the built environment and physical activity that bears further investigation. However, it is difficult to sort out which characteristics of the built environment have the strongest association. Nor does the literature illuminate the strength of the associations or the populations affected. (For example, an environmental attribute may be strongly associated with higher levels of physical activity but affect only a small subpopulation; conversely, the environmental attribute may have a small association but affect a large population.) More important, as of this writing, the evidence falls short of establishing causal connections.

Nevertheless, the literature provides preliminary evidence that some characteristics of the built environment may affect physical activity levels, or at least certain types of physical activity (e.g., destination-oriented travel or recreational physical activity).

These characteristics include certain land use measures (e.g., density, diversity of uses), accessibility, certain design features, and certain aspects of the transportation infrastructure (sidewalks in particular). Feeling safe and secure from crime and traffic, although obviously not a physical attribute of the built environment, was found to be closely linked to the decision to be physically active for many population groups—women, including minorities; children; and older adults—and thus warrants further investigation. Personal attitudes, motivation, and social support systems were also found to be critical for physical activity and, in the limited number of studies that included these variables, more important than the physical environment as motivating influences. Thus, the evidence to date suggests that a supportive built environment alone is not sufficient to influence physical activity but plays a facilitating role.

The very limited evidence from the handful of studies that addressed causal connections between the built environment and physical activity suggests a complex relationship. When individual attitudes and residential location preferences are taken into account, the autonomous effects of the built environment (e.g., walkability) on physical activity behavior are often exhibited, but much less strongly and in a more nuanced way. Research that attempts to test causal connections in a wide range of settings is important in advancing the understanding of these effects.

6

Current State of Knowledge

Understanding how the built environment may affect physical activity is a relatively new but rapidly expanding field of inquiry. The literature comes primarily from two fields: urban planning (travel behavior) and public health (physical activity).[1] The former has focused largely on automobile travel but has also explored walking and cycling as modes of travel. The physical activity literature has focused on the personal and social determinants of physically active behavior and on the intensity and the amount of physical activity, with less attention to the type or location of that activity (Handy 2004). Neither field has had a long history of examining the role of the built environment as a determinant of physical activity (Handy 2004).

In this chapter, the empirical evidence on the relationship between the built environment and physical activity is reviewed. The chapter begins with an overview of the literature and then summarizes the evidence by drawing on studies from both the travel behavior and physical activity fields. Where possible, the results are further analyzed to highlight the role of sociodemographic factors, geographic scale, and such mediating variables as safety and security and time. The studies reviewed are primarily cross-sectional, but the results of a few studies whose research designs are more conducive to drawing causal inferences are also discussed. The final section summarizes knowledge gaps revealed by this review.

---

[1] This chapter draws heavily on a literature review and paper commissioned by the committee (Handy 2004).

151

OVERVIEW OF THE LITERATURE

The literature review conducted for this study encompassed 22 studies from the fields of urban planning/travel behavior and 28 studies from the fields of public health/physical activity (Handy 2004). It drew heavily on recently published reviews of studies supplemented with additional studies known to the committee or Handy or published more recently. International studies were included, although the committee recognizes that the social and environmental determinants of physically active behavior may not be fully comparable with nor the results transferable to the situation in the United States. The committee acknowledges the contribution of international scholars and the importance of international collaboration on research linking the built environment and physical activity. At the same time, it cautions the reader that the policy relevance of the experience in other countries for the United States should be examined with care. Differences in land use and transportation patterns (e.g., lower densities, lower transit use, and greater reliance on the automobile in most U.S. metropolitan areas) and dissimilar regulatory and institutional arrangements (e.g., local rather than central control over land use and zoning policies) may limit the applicability of international experience to the United States (TRB 2001). For example, the experience of Australia and Canada, where land use densities and travel patterns are more similar to those of the United States, may have more relevance and transferability than the experience of many more densely populated and transit-oriented European countries.

Handy's (2004) selection of studies for review in her commissioned paper reflects her subjective assessment of the suitability and relevance of the research. She notes that a detailed evaluation of the quality of execution of each study, using criteria such as those employed by the Task Force on Community Preventive Services, was beyond the scope and resources of the review (Handy 2004).[2]

---

[2] The reader is directed to the following references for a thorough discussion of the evidence-based methods used in preparation of the task force's Guide to Community Preventive Services: Briss et al. 2000 and Carande-Kulis et al. 2000.

In fact, a task force review of environmental interventions to promote physical activity is under way but has not yet been completed.[3] The findings and conclusions presented in this chapter reflect the committee's judgment, although, with few exceptions, that judgment agrees with Handy's assessment.

The vast majority of the studies reviewed use a cross-sectional design; that is, they examine outcomes (i.e., levels of physical activity) at a particular point in time as a function of explanatory variables (i.e., characteristics of the built environment that vary by neighborhood or region). As discussed in Chapter 5, this design enables researchers to draw correlations between variables of interest and isolate those that are statistically significant but not to demonstrate causality.

The review in this chapter should not be viewed as exhaustive but as illustrative of the research completed and under way to date. The field is growing rapidly, more interdisciplinary work is being conducted, and new studies and research results are emerging.

REVIEW OF FINDINGS

Findings from the Travel Behavior Literature

The focus of these studies is on destination-oriented walking trips and nonmotorized travel rather than on walking and cycling for recreation and exercise. As noted, nearly all the studies are cross-sectional, and many control for socioeconomic variables—household size, income, automobile ownership, age, gender, race, employment status—drawn primarily from travel diary data. Two studies incorporate attitudinal factors as control variables, including attitudes about transportation and lifestyle preferences (Kitamura et al. 1997; Bagley and Mokhtarian 2002). Measures of the built environment include population and employment density,

---

[3] Part of the review that deals primarily with work site interventions (e.g., industrial plants, universities, and federal agencies) and related informational outreach programs has been completed (Kahn et al. 2002), and the results are discussed in the subsequent section under "Building or Site Level."

land use mix or diversity of land uses, and design (e.g., shade, scenery, presence of attractive stores and houses), features that have been characterized as the three D's of land use—density, diversity, and design (Cervero and Kockelman 1997). Other measures include transportation infrastructure (e.g., presence and continuity of sidewalks), street pattern (e.g., grid, cul-de-sac) and connectivity, presence of bicycle paths, neighborhood type (e.g., traditional versus suburban planned unit development), and accessibility (e.g., distances to destinations or numbers of destinations within a specified distance).

Although it is difficult to summarize the results of these studies in view of the breadth of measures considered, inspection of the study findings (see Handy 2004, Table 3-4, and Table 6-1, pp. 174–189 in this report) suggests that certain measures are positively (or negatively) correlated with walking or cycling for travel.[4] Land use correlates include a few density measures—population, employment, and retail density—and diversity of land uses. All are positively correlated with nonmotorized travel (i.e., the greater the density of population, employment, stores, and mix of land uses, the greater is the number of walking and other nonmotorized trips). Predictably, access (i.e., distance to nearest destination), another land use measure, is negatively correlated with nonmotorized travel in several studies. A grid street network and presence and extent of sidewalks are the primary transportation-related correlates, both being positively correlated with nonmotorized travel. Design features, with the exception of those of commercial areas, are insignificant, but only four studies examine the effect of such features. Certain neighborhood types—traditional,[5] transit-served, and walkable—are positively correlated with walking and nonmotorized travel. The results are difficult to interpret, however, because of the lack of specificity about the characteristics of these neighborhoods.

---

[4] The pluses and minuses in the tables represent results that are statistically significant. The level of significance (e.g., 5 percent, 1 percent) varies from study to study and is not noted.

[5] Traditional neighborhoods are characterized by a people-oriented, small-town scale with such features as sidewalks and front porches, which have been emulated in neotraditional or new-urbanist developments.

Findings from the Physical Activity Literature

The focus of these studies is on walking, primarily for exercise and recreation; other types of physical activity (e.g., vigorous or moderate-intensity exercise, leisure-time physical activity other than walking); and total physical activity (distinguishing between those who are active and inactive or who do and do not meet recommended levels of physical activity). Measures of the built environment used in these studies cover a breadth of variables that differ considerably from those used in the travel behavior literature. They often include perceptual characteristics—perceived safety, aesthetics and other neighborhood characteristics, and accessibility—rather than objective measures. Where objective measures are used, they fall into many of the same categories as in the travel behavior literature, such as accessibility, design, neighborhood type, and infrastructure for nonmotorized transportation. However, the destinations are most often trails, bicycle paths, or recreation centers rather than the more utilitarian destinations in the travel behavior literature (e.g., shopping, transit stations).

Drawing on ecological models, many of these studies include information about individual attitudes and intentions regarding physical activity (e.g., self-consciousness about appearance) and about the social as well as the physical environment (e.g., club membership, engaging in physical activity with another). Thus, these studies are able to assess the relative importance of all these factors in the decision to be physically active. Most of the studies also control for more typical socioeconomic variables, such as age, gender, race, ethnicity, educational level, marital status, employment status, and income level.

With regard to effects of the built environment, the study results reveal that a few measures are significantly correlated with physical activity (see Handy 2004, Table 3-7, and Table 6-2, pp. 190–209 in this report). For example, subjective measures of accessibility are positively correlated with several types of physical activity in a number of studies. Likewise, neighborhood characteristics, identified by both subjective and objective measures such as presence of sidewalks, enjoyable scenery, and seeing others exercising, are positively correlated with walking and total physical activity. The importance of subjective perceptions of neighborhood character-istics is not surprising in view of trip purpose in these studies, which is often for leisure or recreation rather than for destination-oriented travel. Notably absent, however, are strong associations between measures of perceived safety, design, and diversity of land uses and physical activity.

Summary Assessment

The existing literature approaches the relationship between the built environment and physical activity from a broad range of perspectives, areas of expertise, and measures of the variables of interest. The study results provide a growing body of evidence that shows an association between the built environment and physical activity. That having been said, it is difficult—perhaps because of the diversity of the literature—to sort out which char-acteristics of the built environment have the strongest association. Nevertheless, the study results reveal some patterns that suggest opportunities for further investigation.

Land Use

Population, employment, and land use density and mix/diversity are positively correlated with walking in the transportation literature. In the physical activity literature, fewer studies were found that exam-ine land use measures. Land use diversity (one study) was positively correlated with walking, and density of pay and free facilities (one study) was positively correlated with total physical activity levels.

The characteristic of land use density is a good example of the complexities involved in linking the design of the built environment to travel behavior, such as walking in the neighborhood or walk-ing to access transit. Several studies, for example, explored the link between transit use, development density, and urban design (Pushkarev and Zupan 1977; Messenger and Ewing 1996; Frank and Pivo 1994). They found that as density increased at both trip origin and destination, transit use rose, access by walking increased, and automobile use declined. Other analyses have shown that, although more compact development supports more walking and transit use, automobile ownership and travel patterns also reflect differences in the household characteristics and income of persons living at different density levels (Dunphy and Fisher 1996; Schimek 1996). When these factors are controlled for, the independent effect of density becomes far less robust. Moreover, the density thresholds needed to support transit are reached only in the most heavily populated central cities of U.S. metropolitan areas (TRB 1995). Density may well be a proxy for other variables, such as demographics, distance, car ownership levels, and transit service quality (Boarnet and Crane 2001). In her literature review for the committee, Handy (2004) notes that in studies that tested the significance of measures of both density and accessibility, the latter were significant, while the former were not. Indeed, density may serve as a proxy for accessibility, which provides a more direct explanation for travel behavior.

Accessibility
Typically measured as distance from destinations or facilities, accessibility is significantly correlated with physical activity in studies from both the travel behavior and physical activity literatures. In the former, distance from the nearest destinations, such as stores, bus stops, and parks, emerges as a significant correlate of nonmotorized trips in general and of shopping and school trips in particular. Longer distances discourage all travel, but especially nonmotorized. In the physical activity literature, both perceived and objective measures of proximity and convenience of facilities, ranging from exercise equipment at home, to bicycle paths and trails, to parks, to local shopping and transit stops, are significantly and positively correlated with walking, other forms of exercise and recreation, and total physical activity.

The importance of good access to and convenience of facilities and destinations in the decision to be physically active is certainly plausible from a theoretical perspective. As discussed in Chapter 4, reducing the cost of a desired behavior—in this case by increasing the closeness and convenience of trip destinations—helps encourage the desired behavior.

Design

The evidence for a correlation of design features and aesthetic characteristics of neighborhoods with physical activity is more limited. Design variables, such as neighborhood aesthetics and enjoyable scenery, emerge most strongly in the physical activity literature as significant correlates of physical activity, particularly walking. The one statistically significant result in the travel behavior literature is the positive correlation of design variables with walking trips for shopping. Handy et al. (1998) found that positive perceptions about shade, scenery, traffic, people, safety, and walking incentive and comfort were positively correlated with numbers of walking trips to neighborhood commercial areas.

These limited findings about the importance of design could reflect either the small number of studies that examined these variables, particularly in the travel behavior literature, or poorly specified measures of design. They could also signal the lack of a significant relationship between design and physical activity, or a relationship that may depend on the particular type of physical activity involved. Handy (2004) suggests the latter and concludes that design measures may be a more important influence on walking for recreation and exercise than on destination-oriented travel. Indeed, another review of the literature, drawing on a different set of studies, arrived at much the same conclusion (Humpel et al. 2002). Both reviewers, however, conclude that more research is needed to determine which aspects of design may matter and how they are related to different types of physical activity.

Transportation Infrastructure

The presence of sidewalks emerges in both literatures as a significant correlate of walking and nonmotorized travel. Other correlated transportation infrastructure measures include the proportion of streets with sidewalks and the percentage of the road network having a grid pattern. Some additional evidence exists that the condition of sidewalks is important to physical activity (Sharpe et al. 2004; De Bourdeaudhuij et al. 2003; Hoechner et al., in press). Senior citizens, in particular, may find uneven and cracked sidewalks barriers to walking because of the risk of falls (Loukaitou-Sideris 2004).

Attitudes and Motivation

The limited number of studies that included individual and interpersonal factors found them to be more important than the physical environment in explaining levels of walking and other forms of physical activity (Kitamura et al. 1997; Bagley and Mokhtarian 2002; Giles-Corti and Donovan 2002b). For example, Handy (1996a) and Moudon et al. (1997) found high levels of walking in suburban areas even though these areas had been rated relatively low in terms of walkability. Thus the built environment may not be that important to those who are highly motivated to walk (Handy 2004). At the other end of the spectrum, a more appealing physical environment may not make a difference to those who have little motivation to walk or engage in other forms of physical activity. For many who fall between these two extremes, however, the built environment can facilitate or constrain physical activity. Handy (2004) concludes, and the committee concurs, that a supportive built environment alone is not sufficient to influence physical activity; nevertheless, it can play a facilitating role.

ANALYSIS OF FINDINGS

Effects of the Built Environment on Different Socioeconomic Groups

Data on physical activity levels of the adult population from the large public health surveys discussed in Chapter 2 indicate that activity levels decrease with age and are lower among women, ethnic and racial minorities, those with less education and low income levels, the disabled, and those living in the southeastern region of the United States (CDC 2003). The committee had hoped to examine the results of the literature review conducted for this study according to various socioeconomic groups to understand how characteristics of the built environment may affect the propensity of these groups to be physically active. Very little could be gleaned on this question, however. This is not surprising given that the results for the general population, with some exceptions, show little consistency in the effects of the various environmental characteristics studied.

An examination of the results of the physical activity literature from the perspective of demographic differences is a good case in point. Of the 28 studies in this literature reviewed by Handy (2004), only nine describe the relationship between the built environment and physical activity separately for some demographic characteristic. Few coherent patterns emerge from the analyses. Seeing others exercising was positively associated with physical activity for African Americans, Hispanics, and rural women (King et al. 2000; Eyler et al. 2003; Wilcox et al. 2000). Physical activity was lower among racial and ethnic minorities who perceived their neighborhood to be unsafe and among older men and women (aged ≥65 years) (CDC 1999). Gender differences are more difficult to interpret. For example, walking and moderate activity among women were positively correlated with diversity of land use, ease of walking to a transit stop, access to local shopping, and emotional satisfaction with a neighborhood, but not with presence of sidewalks or satisfaction with neighborhood services (De Bourdeaudhuij et al. 2003).

Effects of the Built Environment at Different Geographic Scales

The role of the built environment can affect the propensity to be physically active at many geographic scales (the building or site level, the neighborhood, and the region) (see Figure 1-2 in Chapter 1). In general, the issue of geographic scale is underexamined in the recent literature (Boarnet 2004).

Building or Site Level

Little is known about how the design of buildings and their sites may influence physical activity (Zimring et al. 2004), which is why the committee did not focus more of its investigation at this scale. Yet most Americans spend the majority of their day in and around buildings—at home, work, or school. This suggests that these locations can provide important opportunities to be physically active.

The form of buildings and sites is thought to affect physical activity at several spatial scales. These include building elements, such as the layout of stairs and exercise rooms; overall building design; and site selection and design, which comprise connectivity between buildings, connectivity of buildings to the edge of the site, and proximity to off-site amenities (Zimring et al. 2004).

Very limited data could be found on physical activity at home. Two studies included in Handy's (2004) review found that having home exercise equipment was positively correlated with vigorous exercise (De Bourdeaudhuij et al. 2003; Sallis et al. 1989). Workplaces are another important but understudied location for physical activity. Stair use provides a low-cost way to integrate physical activity into the daily routine, and there is some limited evidence that interventions to increase workplace stair use (e.g., motivational signs and music in the stairwell) can be effective, although the duration of the effect is unclear (Kerr et al. 2004). Other, more costly interventions, mainly at work sites (e.g., equipment in fitness centers or community centers, creation of walking trails), in conjunction with informational programs, were found to be effective in increasing physical activity (Kahn et al. 2002). The workplace can also be an important base for walking trips, depending on the location of the building and the site layout. An analysis of trip linkage patterns, for example, found that the highest percentage of non-work-related trips involving physical activity are accounted for by walking to and from the workplace before, during, and after work (Wegmann and Jang 1998). Connectivity between buildings and shelter from the elements, placement of parking, and availability of amenities (walking or running trails in suburban, campuslike office complexes and presence of stores and other desirable destinations near urban office buildings) could encourage more such walking trips (Zimring et al. 2004). Company interest in promoting physical activity can pay off because a healthy workforce reduces health care costs (see Chapter 2).

Neighborhood Level

To date, most of the literature has focused on environmental determinants of physical activity at the neighborhood level, and this is appropriate. The neighborhood provides opportunities for all types of physical activity. Indeed, in a recent survey of U.S. adults— the U.S. Physical Activity Study—approximately two-thirds of respondents identified neighborhood streets as the setting where they engage in physical activity (Brownson et al. 2001). Walking is identified as the most common physical activity, reported by 20 percent of Americans (Ross 2000).

The attributes of the neighborhood built environment that may affect walking and other forms of physical activity have already been discussed. Many of these characteristics, such as the presence of sidewalks, aesthetics and other design features, and convenient access to local shopping and parks, are related primarily to physical activity within the neighborhood, including both destination-oriented travel and physical activity for exercise and recreation. These characteristics are unlikely to affect mode choice for many trips out of the neighborhood, such as commuting or traveling to a regional shopping center.

Regional Level

Another notable gap in the literature is consideration of the effect of the built environment on physical activity at scales larger than the neighborhood. Although many of the micro-scale characteristics of the neighborhood would not matter at the regional level, at least one characteristic—accessibility—would. As discussed above, accessibility can influence mode choice. Longer distances between destinations, for example, often tip the balance in favor of the speed and convenience of automobile travel. Good accessibility can also affect destination choice by drawing residents out of the neighborhood and potentially providing other opportunities for recreation and exercise. Such trade-offs and possible substitutions between physical activity within and outside of neighborhoods can be studied only at a regional scale.

Role of Mediating Variables

The relationship between the built environment and physical activity operates through many mediating variables, including socioeconomic characteristics, personal attitudes and motivation, cognitive and behavioral skills, safety and security, and time. Individual characteristics, attitudes, and skills have been discussed earlier in this chapter and in Chapter 4; the effects of safety and security and time are discussed here.

Safety and Security
Intuitively, it is expected that if individuals perceived their environment to be unsafe, they would not be inclined to risk exposure to harm by walking or cycling or would do so only for necessary trips. Because of the likely influence of safety and security on physical activity levels, the committee commissioned a separate paper to review the literature on this topic (Loukaitou-Sideris 2004).

The paper begins by distinguishing among the primary sources of danger for pedestrians and cyclists. The main human-caused sources are crime and vehicular traffic, while the main environmental sources are roadway design (wide, heavily trafficked streets with limited or no accommodation for pedestrians and cyclists), infrastructure condition (e.g., broken and uneven sidewalks), and unattended dogs. These distinctions are important because each source of danger is related to different safety concerns, which may in turn determine which characteristics of the built environment act to inhibit or encourage physically active behavior.

Despite the presumed importance of safety and security to levels of physical activity, neither Loukaitou-Sideris (2004) nor Handy (2004), who also examined safety as a perceived neighborhood characteristic by drawing on a somewhat different group of studies, found evidence for a strong correlation. Loukaitou-Sideris (2004) suggests several reasons for this. First, a number of studies combined safety with other physical attributes in a composite measure that may have obscured the independent effect of safety. In other studies, there was little variation in the environment in which safety effects were examined; these studies were conducted in either unsafe neighborhoods or neighborhoods where safety was not a major concern and thus did not involve a mix of neighborhoods from a safety perspective. Finally, the studies did not always distinguish among different types of safety (e.g., crime, traffic), which, as discussed above, can obscure significant findings.

Personal Safety The results of studies that focused on subpopulations of women, children, and older adults or did a better job of identifying neighborhood environmental characteristics associated with safety and physical activity show a stronger positive correlation between real and perceived dangers to personal safety and sedentary lifestyles (Loukaitou-Sideris 2004). For example, several studies have found that crime and fear of crime are barriers to exercising and being physically active outdoors for women, particularly minority women (CDC 2003; King et al. 2000). These results have been confirmed in numerous focus groups for urban African American women, American Indian women, and Latina immigrant women (Eyler et al. 1998; Wilbur et al. 2002; Young et al. 2002; Thompson et al. 2002; Evenson et al. 2002). Likewise, parental concerns about safety curtail children's activity levels, from use of public spaces such as parks and other play spaces (Valentine and McKendrick 1997; Sallis, McKenzie, et al. 1997; Sallis et al. 1998) to participation in nonschool sports programs (Seefeldt et al. 2002). Older adults are another vulnerable group. Numerous studies have found that older adults may restrict their activity because of concern about personal safety (CDC 1999; Booth et al. 2000). The impact of safety on the behavior of the elderly was dramatically illustrated in a comparative study of mortality rates in two Chicago neighborhoods during the July 1995 heat wave (Klinenberg 2002). The author attributes the higher mortality rates in the neighborhood with abandoned buildings, high rates of violent crime, and limited social support systems in part to the physical characteristics of that community: elderly residents were isolated and afraid to venture forth to seek cooler shelter.

A recent study of urban youth that includes carefully collected data on local socioeconomic and physical characteristics for 80 Chicago neighborhoods found that lack of community safety and measures of social (public intoxication, selling drugs, prostitution) but not physical (graffiti, abandoned cars, needles and syringes) disorder were associated with lower levels of recreational physical activity. These effects remained significant after differences in neighborhood socioeconomic characteristics where taken into account (Molnar et al. 2004).

Traffic Safety Approximately 5,400 pedestrians and cyclists were killed in the United States in 2003, and an additional 116,000 were injured, although these numbers have been declining over time (NCSA 2003a; NCSA 2003b). Children and the elderly are the most vulnerable to pedestrian–automobile collisions—children in terms of injuries and older adults in terms of fatalities (Loukaitou-Sideris 2004). In 2003, children under the age of 16 made up 22 percent of the population, and although they represented only 9 percent of pedestrians killed in crashes, they accounted for 27 percent of pedestrians injured. Older adults (aged ≥70) represented 9 percent of the population but accounted for 16 percent of pedestrian fatalities (NCSA 2003b). With respect to cyclists, the most vulnerable age group was 10- to 15-year-olds, who accounted for less than 9 percent of the population but 16 percent of those killed in crashes (NCSA 2003a).

Although pedestrian and cyclist fatalities are the result of many factors (e.g., motorist behavior; alcohol involvement of drivers, pedestrians, and cyclists), characteristics of the built environment and the transportation infrastructure are part of the story. Most pedestrian–automobile collisions involving children happen in residential areas near a child's home (Sharples et al. 1990) or on the journey to school because exposure is higher in these locations. Child pedestrian injuries appear to be higher in poor neighborhoods, for example, where children play in the streets, often because they lack access to other safe play spaces (Corless and Ohland 1999).

Lack of sidewalks and protected areas for walking and cycling to school can contribute to high levels of pedestrian collisions. Although walking and cycling represent a small fraction of all school trips (less than 20 percent), these modes have the highest fatality and injury rates on a per mile basis (TRB 2002).[6] The safety of older adult pedestrians is also compromised by short traffic signal timing and wide streets with inadequate median "safe havens" (Dorfman 1997). The safety of the pedestrian population of all ages appears to be inversely associated with high traffic speeds (Jacobsen et al. 2000), number of miles of major arterial streets in a neighborhood (Levine et al. 1994), poorly located bus stops and crosswalks (Walgren 1998), and poor lighting.

Few studies were found that directly examine the effect of traffic, either real or perceived, on levels of walking and cycling. Handy

---

[6] A study by the Santa Ana Unified School District in California, cited by Loukaitou-Sideris (2004), found that more than half the city's 72 pedestrian–automobile collisions during the first 6 months of 1998 involved children walking near schools (*Los Angeles Times* 1999).

(1996b) found that the perception of safety, which, as noted, is associated with the decision to walk, is influenced by the speed of automobile traffic. In the surveys reviewed in Chapter 4, parents mentioned traffic danger as a barrier to their children's walking or cycling more to school (Dellinger and Staunton 2002; BR&S 2003). Clearly, efforts to increase physical activity by encouraging more walking and cycling need to be undertaken with care. Raising exposure levels can increase the risk of injury from traffic unless mitigation measures are taken.[7]

Time

The role of time in total physical activity levels is potentially important but poorly understood. Lack of time is often cited as a reason for not being more physically active, and modern life is time-pressured for many. Yet the time-use data cited in Chapter 3 suggest that labor-saving devices, particularly in the home, have freed up more discretionary time for many Americans. The figures on television watching alone—about 3 hours a day for the average U.S. adult—suggest that making time for physical activity is a matter of choice for many Americans.

Recognizing how time affects activity choices should be helpful in understanding the decisions and trade-offs individuals make with regard to physical activity. Individuals may have a time budget for active pursuits and may substitute one type of physical activity for another (e.g., cycling to work rather than exercising at home or at a gym).

Understanding how individuals allocate their time over the course of a day is also important in considering possible interventions. Opportunities for encouraging physical activity exist in many settings—at home, at work, at school, in travel, and in leisure. Rebuilding physical activity into the daily routine may not be so difficult if the goal is to ensure that Americans accumulate at least

---

[7] A recent study, however, provides a counterexample. Researchers analyzed the relationship between the rates of pedestrian and bicycle activity and the number of times pedestrians or cyclists were hit by cars. They found that, in most cases, the risk of collision went down as pedestrian and bicycle activity increased. The author hypothesizes that motorists may drive more carefully in the presence of large numbers of pedestrians and cyclists (Jacobsen 2003).

30 minutes a day of moderate-intensity activity in increments of 10 minutes on most days of the week. Small changes in activity levels in a number of different locations could probably accomplish this objective.

Evidence for Causality

The correlation between certain characteristics of the built environment and higher levels of physical activity does not prove that the built environment caused the physical activity. As noted in Chapter 5, for example, the issue of self-selection bias must be addressed: individual preferences for being physically active may determine the decision to live in a walking- and cycling-friendly environment and account for some or all of the higher levels of physical activity often observed in these neighborhoods. The research designs of a handful of studies enable some analysis of the complex relationships among individual preferences, the built environment, and physical activity levels. Various possible research designs that can lay the foundation for treating the complexities of cause-and-effect relationships are outlined in Chapter 5. They include longitudinal studies using time-series data, case-control cross-sectional studies, and other natural experiments.

Several researchers have used instrumental variable techniques to examine the potential effect of self-selection bias.[8] Boarnet and Sarmiento (1998) and Greenwald and Boarnet (2001) used such

---

[8] In technical terms, the self-selection issue is a manifestation of "endogeneity bias." Ordinary least-squares regression analysis requires that observed explanatory variables be deterministic (not random) and uncorrelated with any unobserved explanatory variables (captured by the error term of the equation). When that requirement is violated, as it is when an explanatory variable itself is a nondeterministic function of other variables in the model, the resulting coefficient estimates are biased. In the present case, the explanatory variable residential location is apt to be determined partly by variables such as attitudes toward travel—variables that are also likely to be observed or unobserved influences on travel behavior itself. Thus, residential location is endogenous. The instrumental variables technique treats this problem by purging the endogenous variable (residential location) of its correlation with other variables in the equation for travel behavior. It does so by first estimating residential location as a function of variables not expected to be associated with travel behavior. The estimated value of residential location then meets the requirements for unbiased ordinary least-squares estimation of the equation for travel behavior. See Chapter 5 for more detailed discussion of research methods.

techniques to control for choice of residential location in studying how neotraditional neighborhoods affected nonwork automobile and pedestrian travel, respectively. Their work tested the hypothesis that the land use characteristics of neotraditional developments (e.g., grid street patterns, higher-density housing, mixed uses) would encourage more walking and other types of nonmotorized travel. In both cases, the researchers found that when variables associated with residential location preferences were identified and examined separately from variables associated with the built environment, some, but not all, of the environmental variables ceased to be significantly correlated with nonmotorized travel. For example, Greenwald and Boarnet (2001) found that population density at the block level and a combined measure of pedestrian-friendly characteristics (ease of street crossing, sidewalk continuity, street connectivity, and topography) remained significant predictors of nonwork pedestrian travel after location preferences were taken into account.

Cervero and Duncan (2002) examined mode choice among residents of transit-oriented developments by using nested logit techniques. In this analysis, mode choice was expressed hierarchically as a function of residential location, which in turn was expressed as a function of workplace location. On the basis of conditional probabilities from the nested logit output, an estimated 40 percent of transit mode choice among station-area residents was explained by the decision to reside near transit in the first place.

In one study using the structural equations modeling approach, researchers attempted to separate out the effects of attitudes, residential location choice, and travel behavior in urban and suburban neighborhoods (Bagley and Mokhtarian 2002).[9] A structural equations model of residential location and travel demand that included attitudinal and lifestyle explanatory variables enabled the researchers to analyze both direct and indirect effects, as well as the

---

[9] Structural equations modeling recognizes that causal influences may work in more than one direction; therefore, multiple equations reflecting these causal linkages are simultaneously modeled (hence using a "structural model" rather than a single equation).

possibility of multiple directions of causality.[10] The authors conclude that attitudinal and lifestyle variables had the greatest impact on travel demand among all the explanatory variables; land use characteristics had little independent effect.

Another study, discussed in Chapter 4, compared the commuting patterns of matched and mismatched residents in three neighborhoods in the San Francisco Bay Area (one urban and two suburban) and attempted to separate the effects of household location preferences from those of the spatial characteristics of residential neighborhoods (Schwanen and Mokhtarian 2004).[11] As in the work of Bagley and Mokhtarian (2002), the researchers found that attitudes and lifestyle variables influenced commuting behavior: suburban-minded residents of the urban neighborhood commuted by private vehicle more often than their urban-minded neighbors (although less often than suburban-minded suburban residents). However, the authors did find some evidence that neighborhood structure itself has an autonomous effect on commuting choices. In both studies, the authors acknowledge the limitations of a cross-sectional approach, which prevented their capturing changes in behavior over time.

Krizek (2003) attempted to address such longitudinal changes by examining modifications in travel behavior among those who move from one neighborhood to another. On the basis of data from the Puget Sound Transportation Panel, he examined the travel behavior of a sample of households that had moved between 1989 and 1997 to neighborhoods with higher local accessibility. Regression models were used to predict changes in travel behavior as a function of changes in neighborhood accessibility, while changes in life cycle and regional and workplace accessibility were held constant. Krizek found that residents who moved to

---

[10] The researchers estimated a nine-equation model for residential location (traditional or suburban), attitudes (pro–high density, pro-driving, pro-transit), and travel demand (vehicle miles, transit miles, and walk/bicycle miles) as endogenous variables for a sample of 515 residents of five neighborhoods in the San Francisco Bay Area.

[11] The data for this study came from responses to a mailed questionnaire that solicited information on a variety of travel and related issues. A multinomial logit analysis model was used to analyze the results (Schwanen and Mokhtarian 2004).

neighborhoods with better local accessibility, all else being equal, had significantly reduced vehicle and person miles traveled (VMT and PMT) and number of trips per tour but increased average number of trips. Difference in neighborhood accessibility, however, was not a significant predictor of changes in walking, cycling, and transit use, which suggested that household travel preferences remained fixed despite changes in residential location. The author hypothesizes that households having moved to an area with greater neighborhood accessibility took more trips but reduced their overall VMT and PMT because their destinations were closer to home. The impact on physical activity levels, which is not discussed by the author, is unknown. The author cautions that, although his longitudinal approach represents an advance in understanding the dynamic effects on travel behavior of a change in urban form (i.e., moving from a low- to a high-accessibility neighborhood), it was limited because no attempt was made to control for possible self-selection bias.

Another longitudinal study of the effect of changes in the built environment on nonmotorized travel—a natural-experimental study of the impact of improvements in traffic safety on children walking and cycling to school—was summarized in Chapter 4. The authors (Boarnet et al. 2004) surveyed parents of children and made independent observations of traffic volumes, speeds, and numbers of pedestrians and cyclists to examine the impact of California's Safe Routes to School Program. They found mixed results: improvements in safety conditions had increased the numbers of children walking and cycling to school at some, but not all, sites. The authors conclude that limitations in the before-and-after study design and the relatively short time frame of the study precluded a more definitive assessment but also discuss the merits of natural-experimental research designs (Boarnet et al. 2004).[12]

---

[12] Ideally, for example, baseline activity data should be collected before the intervention occurs. Respondents would then be questioned about changes in activity after the construction projects had been implemented. Boarnet et al. (2004) used a "second-best" retrospective approach. They asked respondents to recall and compare activity levels before and after project implementation (Boarnet 2004).

Another cross-sectional study also followed a natural-experimental research design. The researchers paired two distinctly designed neighborhoods—one a neotraditional neighborhood and the other a conventional suburban development—to observe differences in physical activity behavior (Rodriguez et al. 2005). Household heads were asked to keep a travel diary and complete a written survey. The researchers isolated the variables of interest—the effect of neighborhood form on various measures of physical activity—by matching the neighborhoods on various other characteristics (regional and freeway access, property values, and age of development) and adjusting for individual and household characteristics.[13] The researchers found that levels of walking and cycling were indeed greater in the neotraditional neighborhood, primarily as a result of more in-neighborhood utilitarian trips by non-motorized means. Total levels of physical activity were also greater in the neotraditional neighborhood, but the differences were not statistically significant. The authors note that more walking and cycling among residents of the neotraditional neighborhood appeared to substitute for their physical activity at other locations, because the total levels of physical activity for surveyed households in both neighborhoods were not significantly different. The authors acknowledge the limitations of relying on self-reports of the frequency and location of physical activity, a relatively low response rate that could have biased the results, and limitations on the generalizability of their results to other neighborhoods. However, they raise important issues that merit further investigation, such as the possibility of substitution effects among different types of physical activity and the fact that different attributes of the built environment may be important for different types of physical activity.

Together, the few studies reviewed here provide limited but provocative results concerning the complexity of causal connections between the built environment and physical activity levels.

---

[13] The researchers examined the total amount of physical activity, the location of that activity (i.e., at home, in the neighborhood, outside the neighborhood), and the frequency and duration of all physical activity trips, and they examined recreational and utilitarian physical activity trips separately (Rodriguez et al. 2005).

Those results suggest a far more nuanced relationship than has been investigated in much of the empirical work to date.

KNOWLEDGE GAPS

In its assessment of the empirical evidence to date, the committee identified several areas in which it believes knowledge gaps currently exist. The following discussion of such gaps is not exhaustive, but it covers many of the critical areas in which further research would help clarify the complex relationships between the built environment and physical activity.

Nonresidential Settings

Most empirical research to date on the influences of the built environment on physical activity has focused on residential neighborhoods. Relatively few studies have examined relationships for nonresidential settings. In the transportation field, this is partly because travel surveys are normally conducted at the household level. Given the importance of studying total physical activity levels across all settings, it would be useful to know more about physical activity in such settings as employment centers, shopping malls, mixed-use projects, and schools. Are campus-style office parks (which are a far cry from neotraditional designs) conducive to physical activity? Even though most people reach enclosed shopping malls by car and vast expanses of surface parking are provided, do these facilities promote walking, especially for certain subgroups of the population such as senior citizens? Are the mixed-use profiles of edge cities as inducements to walking offset by the absence of continuous sidewalk networks and pedestrian-unfriendly designs? Do buildings with prominent, well-lit, open staircases encourage physical activity? To what extent do signage, location of common areas, and availability and location of specific services within building complexes influence physical activity levels at work or at school? Expanding research to nonresidential settings would broaden the understanding of relationships over a wide array of built environments and provide important insights into the totality of physically active behaviors.

Self-Selection

Some progress has been made in understanding the effects of self-selection on physical activity, but greater attention needs to be given to designing research that accounts for such influences as peoples' lifestyle preferences and attitudes. The physical activity benefits of pedestrian-friendly designs need to be understood relative to, for example, the benefits of removing barriers to residential self-selection, such as exclusionary zoning or community resistance to infill housing construction. In addition, are opportunities to sort oneself into physical activity–friendly communities similar across socioeconomic groups? Might low-income and minority house-holds face greater barriers to residential self-selection?

Interactive and Mediating Effects

Little research has been conducted to examine how built environments may interact with other policy interventions, such as road user pricing or flexible parking standards, to influence physical activity. Possible synergistic effects need to be explored to provide a stronger foundation for informing public policy. The role of time is another understudied variable that warrants greater attention. To what extent do individuals substitute one type of physical activity for another (e.g., exercise at work for exercise at home or in the neighborhood)? What is the effect on total physical activity levels?

Stratification

Relationships among built environments, policy interventions, and physical activity outcomes likely vary by subpopulation, urban setting, climate, and other contextual factors. Future research needs to use study designs and populations suitable for examining differences in various subgroupings. It is important to determine which environmental design strategies are most beneficial in different settings and in different types of communities, from well-to-do to low-income.

TABLE 6-1 Summary of Existing Research—Travel Behavior Literature

Study	Sampling[a]	Survey	Active Travel Variable
Bagley and Mokhtarian 2002	515 individuals in five neighborhoods in San Francisco Bay Area	1992 three-day travel diary survey	Natural log of walk/bike miles
Black et al. 2001	4,214 parents at 51 selected infant schools in two regions in the United Kingdom	1996 recall survey distributed through schools	Percent walking as usual mode to school
Cervero 1996[c]	42,200 housing units in 11 metropolitan statistical areas; trips as unit of analysis	1985 American Housing Survey, questionnaire on commuting, cross-sectional survey	Choice of walk or bike as principal commute mode
Cervero and Duncan 2003	7,889 trips, trips as unit of analysis	2000 Bay Area Travel Survey, 2-day activity diary survey, cross-sectional	Choice of walking or biking (with variables for weekend trip, recreation/entertainment, eating/meal, social, shopping purposes)

Controls/ Confounders	Built Environment Variable[b]	Results
Age Gender Household size Number of children under 16 Number of vehicles Years lived in Bay Area Lifestyle factors (seven factors) Attitudes (10 factors)	Suburban factor Traditional factor	Not significant
Full-time homemaker Only one car Southern county	Distance to school	Percent walking: –distance (<0.5 mile—89.5% walk, 0.3% bike; 0.5 to 1 mile—66.4% walk, 1.2% bike; 1.1 to 2 miles—27.7% walk, 2.0% bike; >2 miles— 5.5% walk, 0.8% bike) (not statistically tested)
Residence in central city (y/n) Number of autos Household income Highway or railroad or airport within 300 ft (y/n) Public transit adequate in neighborhood (y/n) Distance from home to work	Single-family housing within 300 ft (y/n) Low-rise multifamily housing within 300 ft (y/n) Mid-rise multifamily housing within 300 ft (y/n) High-rise multifamily housing within 300 ft (y/n) Commercial or non-residential building within 300 ft (y/n) Grocery or drugstore between 300 ft and 1 mile (y/n)	Walk/bike choice: –single-family –ratio of single-family to multi-family low-rise +mid-rise multifamily +high-rise multifamily +commercial nearby –grocery or drug between 300 ft and 1 mile (logit model)
Disability Gender Race Auto ownership	Constraints Deterrents: • Trip distance • Slope • Rainfall day of trip • Dark at time of trip • Low-income neighborhood	Choice of walking: –distance –slope –rainfall +land use diversity—origin +weekend trip, recreation/ entertainment, eating/meal, social, or shopping purpose

(continued)

TABLE 6-1 (*continued*) **Summary of Existing Research— Travel Behavior Literature**

Study	Sampling[a]	Survey	Active Travel Variable
Cervero and Gorham 1995[c]	26 neighborhoods, 14 pairs in San Francisco Bay Area, 12 pairs in Los Angeles region	1990 U.S. Census, cross-sectional	Number of walk trips to work Percent walk trips to work
Cervero and Radisch 1996[c]	620 households for nonwork survey, 840 households for work survey in six census tracts in two neighborhoods in East Bay in San Francisco Bay Area	1994 recall mail surveys, one for work trips, one for non-work trips, cross-sectional	Choice of nonauto mode for non-work trips Choice of nonauto mode for work trips
EPA 2003	709 trips to K-12 school, trips as unit of analysis	2001 Gainesville Metropolitan Transportation Planning Organization Survey and 2000 Florida Department	Choice of walking to school Choice of biking to school

Controls/ Confounders	Built Environment Variable[b]	Results
	Characteristics: • Employment accessibility • Ped/bike design at origin • Ped/bike design at destination • Land use diversity— origin • Land use diversity— destination	Choice of biking: −distance −dark +recreation/entertainment or social purpose (logit model)
Neighborhoods matched for income	Transit versus automobile neighborhood	Number of walk trips: +transit neighborhoods (23 to 142 more walk trips per 1,000 households in San Francisco Bay Area; from 1 to 179 more walk trips per 1,000 households in Los Angeles region) Percent walk trips: +transit neighborhoods (1.2 to 13.4 percentage points more walk trips in San Francisco Bay Area, from 1.7 to 24.6 percentage points more walk trips in Los Angeles region)
Household size Vehicles per household Annual salary of respondent	Pedestrian versus automobile neighborhood	Choice of nonauto mode for nonwork trips: +traditional Choice of nonauto mode for work trips: not significant (logit model)
Income Cars per household Driver's license	Overall density (jobs and employment) Commercial floor area ratio Percent of streets with sidewalks Average sidewalk width	Choice of walking: −walk time +sidewalk coverage Choice of biking:a −bike time (logit model)

(*continued*)

TABLE 6-1 (*continued*) **Summary of Existing Research—Travel Behavior Literature**

Study	Sampling[a]	Survey	Active Travel Variable
		of Transportation Survey, 1-day travel diary survey, cross-sectional	
Ewing et al. 1994[c]	163 households from six communities in Palm Beach County, Florida	c. 1994 Palm Beach County, Florida, Travel Survey, 2-day travel diary survey, cross-sectional	Percent walk or bike trips of all trips
Frank and Pivo 1994[c]	1,680 households, weighted to regional total in Puget Sound, Washington, region; census tract as unit of analysis	1989 Puget Sound Transportation Panel survey, 2-day travel diary survey, cross-sectional	Percent walk trips for work trips for census tract Percent walk trips for shopping trips for census tract
Friedman et al. 1994[c]	Selected zones from 550 zones in San Francisco Bay Area	1980 Bay Area Travel Survey, 1-day travel diary survey, cross-sectional	Average number of walk trips per day per household Average number of bicycle trips

Controls/ Confounders	Built Environment Variable[b]	Results
	Street density Pedestrian environment factor Walk time to school Bike time to school	
None	Neighborhood	Percent walk or bike trips: not significant (ANOVA)
Mean age for residents of tract Household type (defined by number of adults and age, share for tract) Driver's license (share for tract) Trips made by employed resident (share of trip ends in tract) Trips made by residents with bus pass (share of trip ends in tract) Trips made by residents with access to less than one vehicle (share of trip ends in tract), mean number of vehicles available per participant ending trip in tract	Gross population density at origin Gross population density at destination Gross employment density at origin Gross employment density at destination Land use mix at origin (entropy measure) Land use mix at destination (entropy measure)	Percent walk trips for work: +employment density at origin +population density at origin +population density at destination +land use mix at origin +land use mix at destination Percent walk trips for shopping: +employment density at trip destination +population density at trip origin +population density at destination (linear regression; 31% and 35% of variation explained)
None	Traditional versus standard suburban communities	Number of walk trips: +traditional (1.06 versus 0.83) Number of bike trips: +traditional (0.35 versus 0.24) Percent walk trips: +traditional (12% versus 8%)

(*continued*)

TABLE 6-1 *(continued)* **Summary of Existing Research—Travel Behavior Literature**

Study	Sampling[a]	Survey	Active Travel Variable
			per day per household Percent walk trips for zone Percent bike trips for zone (all by purpose)
Greenwald and Boarnet 2001	1,091 residents from Portland, Oregon, region	1994 Portland Travel Survey, 2-day travel diary survey, cross-sectional	Number of walk trips in 2 days
Handy 1996a[c]	400 residents in four neighborhoods in San Francisco Bay Area	1992 recall phone survey, cross-sectional	Number of strolling trips per month Percent of residents strolling at least once per month Number of walking trips to commercial area per month Percent of residents walking to commercial area at least once per month
Handy et al. 1998 and Handy and Clifton 2001[c]	1,368 residents in six neighborhoods in Austin, Texas	1994 recall mail survey, cross-sectional	Number of strolling trips per month Number of walking trips to commer-

Controls/ Confounders	Built Environment Variable[b]	Results
		Percent bike trips: +traditional (4% versus 2%) (no statistical testing)
Age Gender Race Income Square of income Number of children under 16 Cars per driver Employees per household Workday	Population density in block group Population density in zip code Retail density in 1-mile grid cell Retail density in zip code Percent of network that is a grid Pedestrian environment factor (three-point scale): ease of street crossing, sidewalk continuity, street connectivity, topography Median walk distance Median walk speed	Number of walk trips: +population density +retail density +percent of network that is a grid +pedestrian environment factor +median walk distance +median walk speed (ordered probit model)
Household type (defined by number of adults, work status)	Traditional versus suburban neighborhood	Average strolling frequency: not significant Percent of residents strolling: not significant Walking trips to commercial area: +traditional (4.8 to 5.7 versus 1.0 to 2.8 walks per month) Percent walking to commercial areas: +traditional (56% to 64% versus 33% to 48%) (ANOVA)
Age Gender Employment status	Network distance to nearest commercial area (using GIS)	Number of strolling trips: +perceived safety +perceived shade +perceived people

(*continued*)

TABLE 6-1 (*continued*) **Summary of Existing Research—Travel Behavior Literature**

Study	Sampling[a]	Survey	Active Travel Variable
			cial area per month
Hanson and Schwab 1987	278 households stratified by life cycle stage in Uppsala, Sweden	1971 Uppsala 35-day travel diary survey, cross-sectional	Percent of all stops by nonmotorized modes Percent of work stops by non-motorized modes
Kitamura et al. 1997[c]	1,380 individuals in five neighbor-hoods in San Francisco Bay Area	1992 three-day travel diary survey	Number of non-motorized trips Percent nonmotor-ized trips for all trips

Controls/ Confounders	Built Environment Variable[b]	Results
Presence of children under age 5 Income Pet to walk	Perceptual factors related to safety, shade, houses, scenery, traffic, people, stores, walking incentive, walking comfort	+Old West Austin neighbor- hood Number of walking trips to commercial areas: −distance +perceived stores +perceived walking incentive +perceived walking comfort +Old West Austin neighbor- hood +strolling frequency (linear re- gression, 15% and 29% of variation explained)
Gender Employment status Automobile availability	Home-based accessi- bility Work-based accessi- bility (number of establishments by 0.5-km intervals, weighted by distance, using Euclidean distance)	Percent of all stops: +home-based accessibility Percent of work stops: +home-based accessibility +work-based accessibility (correlation coefficients)
Age Gender Education level Employment status Homemaker (y/n) Student (y/n) Professional (y/n) Driver's license (y/n) Household size Number of persons over 16 years Number of autos Household income Number of years in Bay Area Apartment/single- family home Attitudes (nine factors)	Study area Macro-scale descrip- tors (y/n): BART access, mixed land use, high density Pedestrian/bicycle facility indicators (y/n): sidewalk, bike path Micro-scale accessi- bility indicators: distance to nearest bus stop, rail sta- tion, grocery store, gas station, park Perceptions of quality of residential neigh- borhood: no reason to move, street pleasant for walk- ing, cycling pleas- ant, good local transit service,	Number of nonmotorized trips: +North San Francisco neighbor- hood +BART access +sidewalk Share of nonmotorized trips: +high density −distance to nearest bus stop −distance to nearest park (linear regression)

(*continued*)

TABLE 6-1 (*continued*) **Summary of Existing Research— Travel Behavior Literature**

Study	Sampling[a]	Survey	Active Travel Variable
Kockelman 1997[c]	9,000 households; trips as unit of analysis	1990 Bay Area Travel Survey, 1-day travel diary survey, cross-sectional	Choice of walk or bike for all trips by adults
Krizek 2000	550 households that moved between 1989 and 1997 in Puget Sound, Washington, region	1989 and 1997 Puget Sound Transportation Panel, 2-day travel diary survey, longitudinal	Percent of trips by alternative mode (transit, walk, bike) Change in percent of trips by alternative mode (transit, walk, bike)

Controls/ Confounders	Built Environment Variable[b]	Results
	enough parking, problems of traffic congestion	
Age Gender Race Household size (members over age 5) Auto ownership Income per household member Driver's license Employment status Professional job	Population density in origin zone, destination zone Employment density in origin zone, destination zone Accessibility (gravity measure, sales and service jobs within 30 minutes by walk mode) in origin zone, destination zone Land use balance (entropy index, six land use types) for zone, mean for all zones within 0.5 mile General land use mix (dissimilarity index, four land use types) Detailed land use mix (dissimilarity index, 11 land use types)	Choice of walk or bike: +accessibility in origin zone +accessibility in destination zone (+0.22 elasticity) +mean nonwork entropy in origin zone +mean entropy in destination zone (+0.23 elasticity) (logit model)
None	LADUF rating: land use mix (number of employees of selected types), density (housing units and persons per square mile), urban form rating (average block area per grid cell); measured for 150-m grid cells, averaged over all grid cells within 0.4 km Change in LADUF rating	Percent of trips by alternative mode: +LADUF (29% in high, 14% in medium, 6% in low LADUF) Change in percent of trips by alternative mode: −move from high to medium LADUF (9.9 percentage points) (*t*-tests)

(continued)

TABLE 6-1 *(continued)* **Summary of Existing Research—Travel Behavior Literature**

Study	Sampling[a]	Survey	Active Travel Variable
Krizek 2003	550 households that moved between 1989 and 1997 in Puget Sound, Washington, region	1989 and 1997 Puget Sound Transportation Panel, 2-day travel diary survey, longitudinal	Percent of trips by walking
McCormack et al. 2001	663 households from throughout region, split into three zones; 300 households in each of three mixed land use neighborhoods, neighborhood as unit of analysis	1989 Puget Sound Transportation Panel, 2-day travel diary survey, 1992 same survey implemented in three selected neighborhoods, cross-sectional	Percent walk trips for shopping trips for neighborhood Percent walk trips for all trips for neighborhood (only walk trips longer than 5 minutes)
McNally and Kulkarni 1997[c]	20 neighborhoods in Orange County, California, neighborhood as unit of analysis	1991 Southern California Association of Governments, 1-day activity diary survey, cross-sectional	Number of walk trips, percent walk trips

Controls/ Confounders	Built Environment Variable[b]	Results
Number of vehicles Number of adults Number of children Number of workers Income	Neighborhood accessibility: density (housing units per acre), land use mix (number of employees of selected types), average block area; measured for 150-m grid cells, averaged over all grid cells within 0.4 km Regional accessibility (gravity measure)	Percent of trips by walking: not significant
None	Straight-line distance to nearest commercial street Neighborhood type	Percent walk trips for shopping trips: –distance to nearest commercial street Percent walk trips for all trips: +walkable neighborhood (17.7 to 18.1 versus 2.0 to 2.8) (no statistical testing)
Income	Traditional neighborhood development, planned unit development, and mixed (classified on the basis of ratio of cul-de-sacs to total intersections, ratio of four-way to total intersections, intersections/acre, ratio of access points to development perimeter, commercial area to total area, population density)	Number of walk trips: not significant Percent walk trips: not significant (ANOVA)

(*continued*)

TABLE 6-1 (*continued*) **Summary of Existing Research—Travel Behavior Literature**

Study	Sampling[a]	Survey	Active Travel Variable
Moudon et al. 1997 and Hess et al. 1999	12 sites in Seattle, Washington, area, controlled for density, site as unit of analysis	c. 1996 observations for 16 hours at entry points across cordons for sites, cross-sectional	Number of pedestrians
Parsons Brinckerhoff Quade and Douglas, Inc., 1993[c]	400 zones in Portland, Oregon	1985 Portland Metro travel survey, 1-day travel diary survey, cross-sectional	Percent walk or bicycle trips (for trips longer than six blocks) for zone

NOTE: ANOVA = analysis of variance; BART = Bay Area Rapid Transit; LADUF = less auto-dependent urban form; PEF = pedestrian environment factor.

[a]Unit of analysis is individual unless otherwise noted.

[b]Built environment variables are objectively measured unless otherwise noted.

[c]Included in Saelens, Sallis, and Frank 2003.

Controls/ Confounders	Built Environment Variable[b]	Results
None	Urban versus suburban neighborhood	Number of pedestrians: +urban neighborhood (38 versus 12 pedestrians per hour per 1,000 residents) (not statistically tested)
None	Pedestrian environment factor (3-point scale): ease of street crossing, sidewalk continuity, street connectivity, topography Residential density Transit access to employment (number of jobs within 30 minutes by transit)	Percent walk or bike trips: +PEF (from 1.4% in low PEF to 9.6% in high PEF to 18.6% in central business district) +residential density (from 2.0% at zero to two households per acre to 10.4% at five or more households per acre) +transit access (from 2.0% at low access to 13.5% at high access) (no statistical testing)

TABLE 6-2   Summary of Existing Research—Physical Activity Literature

Study	Sampling	Survey	Physical Activity Variable
Ball et al. 2001[c]	3,392 adults in Australia	1996 Physical Activity Survey for state of New South Wales, cross-sectional survey	Walking versus not walking for exercise in last 2 weeks
Berrigan and Troiano 2002	14,827 adults 20 years old or older in United States	NHANES III, cross-sectional survey	Walk 1 or more miles 20 or more times per month (y/n) Leisure-time physical activity other than walking 20 or more times per month (y/n)
Booth et al. 2000[c]	402 adults 60 years old and older in Australia	1995 Supplement to the Population Survey Monitor by the Australian Bureau of Statistics, cross-sectional survey	Sufficiently active versus inactive (based on vigorous activities, moderate activities, and walking for exercise, leisure, or recreation)
Brownson et al. 2000	1,269 adults in 17 communities in 12 rural counties in Missouri, modified BRFSS method	1998 cross-sectional phone survey	Used walking trails (y/n, for those with access) Increased walking since using trails (y/n, for those with access)

Controls/ Confounders[a]	Built Environment Variables	Results[b]
Age Gender Education level	Neighborhood aesthetics (5-point scales): neighborhood friendly, local area attractive, pleasant walking near home Convenience to facilities (5-point scales): park/beach within walking distance, cycle path accessible, shops within walking distance	Walking: +neighborhood aesthetics (high 41% more likely to walk than low) +convenience to facilities (high 36% more likely to walk than low) (logistic regression)
Age Gender Race/ethnicity Household income Education Health-related activity limitation Region	Year when home built (<1946, 1946 to 1973, 1974 to present)	Walking: +age of house (<1946 43% more than 1974 to present house; 1946–1973 house 36% more than 1974 to present house) Leisure time physical activity: not significant (logistic regression)
Age Gender Country of birth Marital status Employment status Living situation Attitudes	Exercise equipment at home (y/n) Feel safe walking during day (y/n) Footpaths safe for walking (y/n) Access to facilities (y/n): local exercise hall, recreation center, cycle paths, golf course, gym, park, swimming pool, tennis course, bowling green	Active: +footpaths safe for walking +access to recreation center +access to cycle track +access to golf course +access to park +access to swimming pool (logistic regression)
Age Gender Race/ethnicity Marital status Education level Income	Population of community (<5,500, 5,500 to 10,000, more than 10,000) Trail length (<¼ mile, ¼ to ½ mile, >½ mile) Trail surface (asphalt, chat, woodchips) Distance to trail (<5 miles, 5–10 miles,	Used walking trails: +5,500 to 10,000 population +¼ to ½ mile length −chat surface (versus asphalt) −woodchips surface (versus asphalt) Increased use: −population +trail length −chat surface (versus asphalt)

(*continued*)

TABLE 6-2 *(continued)* **Summary of Existing Research—Physical Activity Literature**

Study	Sampling	Survey	Physical Activity Variable
Brownson et al. 2001	1,818 adults, United States, modified BRFSS sampling plan, oversampling of lower-income individuals	1999–2000 cross-sectional phone survey, questions based on BRFSS, NHI, other surveys	Meeting recommendations for moderate or vigorous activity (y/n)
CDC 1999[c]	12,767 adults in Maryland, Montana, Ohio, Pennsylvania, Virginia	1996 BRFSS, cross-sectional phone survey	Active versus inactive (based on walking, moderate activity, and vigorous activity)
Craig et al. 2002	27 neighborhoods in Canada (totaling 10,983 residents)	1996 Canadian census, cross-sectional survey	Percent of residents walking to work
De Bourdeaudhuij et al. 2003	521 adults in Ghent, Belgium	c. 2002 cross-sectional mail survey using International Physical Activity Questionnaire	Minutes of sitting, walking, moderate-intensity activities, vigorous-intensity activities in last 7 days

Controls/ Confounders[a]	Built Environment Variables	Results[b]
	11–29 miles, 30 or more miles)	–distance to trail (20% to 30% less if 5 or more miles) (logistic regression)
Age Gender Race/ethnicity Household income Education	Places to exercise (y/n): indoors, outdoors Specific access variables (y/n): walk/jog trail, neighborhood streets, park, shopping mall, indoor gym, treadmill Neighborhood character- istics (y/n): sidewalks, enjoyable scenery, heavy traffic, hills, streetlights, un- attended dogs, foul air from cars/factories Personal barriers (y/n): no safe place, bad weather	Meeting recommendations: +places to exercise indoors or outdoors +places to exercise outdoors only +walking/jogging trail +park +indoors gym +treadmill +sidewalks present +enjoyable scenery +heavy traffic +hills (logistic regression)
Gender Race/ethnicity Education level Income	Perception of safety from crime in neighborhood (4-point scale)	Active: +perceived safe from crime in neighborhood
Income University education Poverty Degree of urban- ization (urban, suburban, small urban)	Observations of 18 char- acteristics on 10-point scales; hierarchical lin- ear modeling to create ecologic score for each neighborhood	Percent walking to work: +ecologic score (1-unit increase in score associated with 25 percentage point increase in walking)
Age Gender Education level Employment status Occupation Living situation BMI	Neighborhood variables (3-, 5-, or 7-point scales): residential density (3 items), land use mix/diversity (13), access to local shop- ping (2), ease of walk- ing to transit stop (1), availability of side- walks (1), availability of bike lanes (2), neigh- borhood aesthetics (4),	*Women* Sitting: –perceived safety from crime +land use mix/diversity Walking: +availability of sidewalks Moderate activity: +physical activity equipment in home +satisfaction with neighbor- hood services

(*continued*)

TABLE 6-2 *(continued)* **Summary of Existing Research—Physical Activity Literature**

Study	Sampling	Survey	Physical Activity Variable
Eyler et al. 2003	4,122 women 20 to 50 years old from diverse racial/ethnic groups (white, African American, Latina, and Native American)	2001–2002 Women and Physical Activity Survey, cross-sectional phone and interview survey	Meets recommendations for moderate or vigorous activity versus does not meet Does any physical activity versus does none
Giles-Corti and Donovan 2002a	1,803 adults 18 to 59 years old in Perth, Australia; excluded from study: unemployed, resident	1995–1996 cross-sectional in-person survey	Walking for transport in past 2 weeks (y/n) Walking for recreation in past 2 weeks (y/n)

Controls/ Confounders[a]	Built Environment Variables	Results[b]
	perceived safety from crime (2), perceived safety from traffic (2), connectivity (2), satisfaction with neighborhood services (2), emotional satisfaction with neighborhood (4) Recreational variables (7-point scales or y/n): work site environment (10 items), physical activity equipment at home (13), convenience of physical activity facilities (18)	Vigorous activity: +physical activity equipment in home +convenience of physical activity facilities *Men* Sitting: −emotional satisfaction with neighborhood Walking: +land use mix/diversity +ease of walking to transit stop Moderate activity: +access to local shopping +emotional satisfaction with neighborhood Vigorous activity: +physical activity equipment in home +convenience of physical activity facilities +work site environment
Racial/ethnic group Urban, rural, mixed settings	Traffic (3-point scale) Presence of sidewalks (y/n) Street lighting at night (3-point scale) Presence of unattended dogs (problem/not a problem) Safety from crime (y/n) Places within walking distance (y/n) Places to exercise (y/n)	Meets recommendations: African American, urban: −fair lighting (versus poor) African American, mixed: +presence of sidewalks Native American, mixed: +unattended dogs not a problem White, rural: −fair lighting (versus poor) Does any activity: African American, rural: −very good/good lighting (versus poor) Latina, urban: −light traffic (versus heavy)
Age Gender Number of children under 18 Household income Education level	Access to built facilities (gravity measures by quartile, from GIS): sport and recreation centers, gyms, swimming pools, tennis courts, golf courses	Walking for transport: −high access to beach (38% less) +high perception that neighborhood has lots of traffic (26% more) +sidewalks (65% more)

(continued)

TABLE 6-2 (*continued*) **Summary of Existing Research—Physical Activity Literature**

Study	Sampling	Survey	Physical Activity Variable
	in suburb for less than 1 year, exercised as recommended at work, medical condition likely to affect physical activity, not proficient in English		Walking at recommended levels (y/n, based on 12 or more sessions in 2 weeks totaling 360 minutes or more)
Giles-Corti and Donovan 2002b[c]	1,803 adults 18 to 59 years old in Perth, Australia	1995–1996 cross-sectional in-person survey	Exercising as recommended (y/n, based on walking for recreation and transportation, light-moderate physical activity, vigorous physical activity) Use of facilities (y/n)

Controls/ Confounders[a]	Built Environment Variables	Results[b]
Work outside home (y/n) Personal access to car (y/n) SES of area of residence	Access to natural facilities (gravity measures by quartile, from GIS): attractive public open space, beach, river Physical environment determinant score (sum of three measures, divided into thirds) Perceptions of neighborhood (5-point scale, 11 items, 3 factors): neighborhood attractiveness, safety and interest; social support for walking locally; traffic and traffic hazards Perceptions of (y/n): sidewalks, streets well lit, public transit within walking distance, park within walking distance, shop within walking distance	+shops within walking distance (3 times) +sometimes access to motor vehicle (3.46 times) +no access to motor vehicle (4.13 times) Walking for recreation: +high access to beach (49% more than lower) +perception neighborhood attractive, safe, interesting (49% more) +sidewalks (41% more) Walking as recommended: +high access to public open space (43% more) +perception neighborhood attractive, safe, interesting (50% more) +sidewalks (65% more) +no access to motor vehicle (2.87 times) (logistic regression)
Age Gender Number of children under 18 Household income Education level	Functional (y/n, observed): sidewalk, shop Appeal: type of street, trees (y/n, observed), extent of tree coverage Access to built facilities (gravity measures by quartile, from GIS): sport and recreation centers, gyms, swimming pools, tennis courts, golf courses Access to natural facilities (gravity measures by quartile, from GIS): attractive public open space, beach, river Physical environment determinant score (sum of three measures, divided into thirds)	Exercising as recommended: −second third of access to built facilities relative to top third (29% less likely) +high physical environment score relative to low (43% more likely) Use of attractive open space: +access Use of river: +access Use of swimming pool: +access (logistic regression)

(continued)

TABLE 6-2 (*continued*) **Summary of Existing Research—Physical Activity Literature**

Study	Sampling	Survey	Physical Activity Variable
Giles-Corti and Donovan 2003	1,803 adults 18 to 59 years old in Perth, Australia	1995–1996 cross-sectional in-person survey	Walking at recommended levels (y/n, based on 12 or more sessions in 2 weeks totaling 360 minutes or more)
Hovell et al. 1989[c]	2,053 adults in San Diego	1986 cross-sectional mail survey	Walking for exercise (number of minutes per week)
King et al. 2000[c]	2,912 women 40 years old and older in United States, modified BRFSS approach	1996–1997 U.S. Women's Determinant Study, cross-sectional survey	Active versus underactive versus sedentary over last 2 weeks (based on moderate activity and vigorous activity)

Controls/ Confounders[a]	Built Environment Variables	Results[b]
Age Gender Number of children under 18 Household income Education level	Functional (y/n, observed): sidewalk, shop Appeal: type of street, trees (y/n, observed), extent of tree coverage Access to built facilities (gravity measures by quartile, from GIS): sport and recreation centers, gyms, swimming pools, tennis courts, golf courses Access to natural facilities (gravity measures by quartile, from GIS): attractive public open space, beach, river Physical environment determinant score (sum of three measures, divided into thirds)	Walking at recommended levels: +high physical environment score (2.13 times as likely as low score) +high access to attractive open space (1.47 times as likely as low access) (logistic regression)
Age Gender Education level Smoking Alcohol Diet	Number of exercise-related items at home (10 items, y/n) Number of exercise facilities perceived as convenient (15 items, y/n) Neighborhood environment (scale): safety of exercising in neighborhood, ease of exercising in neighborhood, frequency of seeing others exercising	Walking: +neighborhood environment (linear regression, 12% of variance explained)
Age Race/ethnicity Employment status Marital status Education level Residence (urban/ rural/other)	Presence of (y/n): sidewalks, heavy traffic, hills, streetlights, unattended dogs, enjoyable scenery, frequently see others exercising, high levels of crime Safe to walk or jog alone during the day (5-point scale) Barriers (5-point scale): lack a safe place to exercise, poor weather	Active: +hills +unattended dogs +enjoyable scenery +frequently see others exercising (logistic regression)

(*continued*)

TABLE 6-2 *(continued)* **Summary of Existing Research—
Physical Activity Literature**

Study	Sampling	Survey	Physical Activity Variable
MacDougall et al. 1997[c]	1,765 adults in Adelaide, Australia	1987 cross-sectional mail survey by the South Australia Community Health Research Unit	Moderately active versus inactive (based on moderate activity, vigorous sport, walking for exercise)
Parks et al. 2003	1,818 adults, United States, modified BRFSS sampling plan, oversampling of lower-income individuals	1999–2000 cross-sectional phone survey, questions based on BRFSS, NHI, other surveys	Meets public health recommendations versus insufficient activity or inactive
Powell et al. 2003	4,532 adults in Georgia	2001 Georgia BRFSS	Meets physical activity recommendations
Ross 2000	2,482 adults in Illinois	1995 Survey of Community, Crime and Health, cross-sectional phone survey	Number of days walking per week Number of days of strenuous exercise per week

Controls/ Confounders[a]	Built Environment Variables	Results[b]
Age Education General health Social connections	Satisfaction with recreation facilities (5-point scale) Satisfaction with living environment (5-point scale)	Moderately active: +satisfied with recreation facilities (logistic regression)
Age Race Gender Stratified by urban, suburban, rural and by high and low income	Places to exercise (y/n): walk/jog trail, neighborhood streets, park, shopping mall, indoor gym, treadmill Number of places to exercise (0 to 4) Personal barriers (y/n): no safe place, bad weather	Meets for urban: +walking/jogging trails +park +indoor gym +treadmill +other equipment +number of places Meets for suburban: +walking/jogging trails +indoor gym Meets for rural: +indoor gym +4 places to exercise
None	Some place to walk (y/n): Not home based: public park, school track, gym or fitness center, walking or jogging trail, shopping mall, other place Home based: neighborhood streets or roads, neighborhood sidewalk, treadmill at home	Meeting recommendations: +public park +school track +gym or fitness center +walking or jogging trail +other place +neighborhood streets or roads +neighborhood sidewalk
Age Gender Race Ethnicity Marital status Education Household income Below poverty line Neighborhood poverty, race, ethnicity, and education characteristics	City of Chicago versus suburb of Chicago versus small city versus small town or rural area	Walking: +Chicago versus small town or rural area

(continued)

TABLE 6-2 *(continued)* **Summary of Existing Research— Physical Activity Literature**

Study	Sampling	Survey	Physical Activity Variable
Rutten et al. 2001	3,343 adults, six European countries (Belgium, Finland, Germany, Netherlands, Spain, Switzerland)	MAREPS study, 1997–1998 cross-sectional phone survey	Level of vigorous activity (sedentary, not/somewhat vigorous, vigorous, very vigorous)
Saelens, Sallis, Black, and Chen 2003	107 adults, two neighborhoods in San Diego	c. 2002 cross-sectional mail survey and accelerometers	Moderate-intensity physical activity (minutes during last 7 days) Vigorous-intensity physical activity (minutes during last 7 days) Total physical activity (minutes during last 7 days)
Sallis et al. 1989[c]	1,789 adults in San Diego	c. 1988 cross-sectional mail survey	Frequency of vigorous exercise (times per week for at least 20 minutes with increase in heart rate or breathing)

Controls/ Confounders[a]	Built Environment Variables	Results[b]
None	Perceived physical activity–related opportunities: Residential area offers many opportunities to be physically active (5-point scale) Local clubs and other providers in community offer many opportunities (5-point scale) Community does not do enough for citizens and their physical activity (5-point scale)	From sedentary to not/somewhat vigorous: +perceived physical activity–related opportunities (ANOVA)
Age Education level	High-walkability versus low-walkability neighborhood	Moderate-intensity: +high-walkability (194.8 versus 130.7 minutes) Total physical activity: +high-walkability (210.5 versus 139.9 minutes)
Age Gender Education level Smoking Alcohol Diet	Number of exercise-related items at home (10 items, y/n) Number of exercise facilities perceived as convenient (15 items, y/n) Neighborhood environment (scale): safety of exercising in neighborhood, ease of exercising in neighborhood, frequency of seeing others exercising Barriers (5-point frequency scale): lack of equipment, lack of facilities, lack of good weather	Vigorous exercise: +home equipment (linear regression; 27% of variation explained with all variables included)

(continued)

TABLE 6-2 (*continued*) **Summary of Existing Research— Physical Activity Literature**

Study	Sampling	Survey	Physical Activity Variable
Sallis et al. 1990[c]	2,053 adults with mean of 48 years in San Diego		Sedentary versus exerciser (based on three or more exercise sessions per week)
Sallis et al. 1992[c]	1,719 adults in San Diego	Prospective study: follow-up to Sallis et al. 1989; mail survey	Frequency of vigorous exercise (times per week for at least 20 minutes with increase in heart rate or breathing) Change in vigorous exercise over 24 months
Sallis, Johnson et al. 1997[c]	110 college students with mean age 20.6 in San Diego	c. 1996 survey administered through college class	Walking for exercise (minutes/week) Strength exercise (days/week) Vigorous exercise (days/week)

Controls/ Confounders[a]	Built Environment Variables	Results[b]
Age Education level Income	Density of pay and free facilities	Exerciser: +density of pay facilities
Age Gender Education level Income Race/ethnicity Marital status Smoking	Number of exercise-related items at home (10 items, y/n) Number of exercise facilities perceived as convenient (15 items, y/n) Neighborhood environment (scale): safety of exercising in neighborhood, ease of exercising in neighborhood, frequency of seeing others exercising Barriers (5-point frequency scale): lack of equipment, lack of facilities, lack of good weather	Change in vigorous activity in sedentary men: −neighborhood environment (linear regression)
	Exercise facilities in home (y/n, 15 items) Neighborhood environment (sum of three items): presence of (y/n): sidewalks, heavy traffic, hills, streetlights, dogs unattended, enjoyable scenery, crime; rating neighborhood as residential, commercial, or mixed; safe for walking during day (5-point scale) Convenient facilities: places to exercise on a frequently traveled route or within 5-minute walk (y/n, 18 places)	Walking for exercise: not significant Strength exercise: +home equipment Vigorous exercise: not significant (linear regression)

(*continued*)

TABLE 6-2 *(continued)* **Summary of Existing Research— Physical Activity Literature**

Study	Sampling	Survey	Physical Activity Variable
Shaw et al. 1991[c]	14,674 adults 18 to 69 years old in Canada who wished to participate in more physical activity	1983 Canada Fitness Survey, cross-sectional survey	Participation in 35 recreational activities (hours per week)
Stahl et al. 2001[c]	3,343 adults, 6 European countries (Belgium, Finland, Germany, Netherlands, Spain, Switzerland)	MAREPS study, 1997–1998 cross-sectional phone survey	Active versus inactive (based on participation in any gymnastics, physical activity, or sports)
Troped et al. 2001[c]	413 adults with mean age 51 years in Arlington, Massachusetts	1998 cross-sectional mail survey	Use versus nonuse of bikeway
Wilcox et al. 2000[c]	2,912 women 40 years old and older in United States, modified	1996–1997 U.S. Women's Determinant Study, cross-	Active versus underactive versus sedentary over last 2 weeks

Controls/ Confounders[a]	Built Environment Variables	Results[b]
Gender	No facilities nearby (y/n) Available facilities are inadequate (y/n)	Participation for women: +no facilities nearby +available facilities inadequate Participation for men: +available facilities inadequate (ANOVA)

Age
Gender
Education level
Country
	Local opportunity scale
	  (5-point scales): area
	  offers many opportuni-
	  ties to be active, local
	  clubs and other
	  providers offer many
	  opportunities, commu-
	  nity does not do
	  enough for citizens and
	  their physical activity
		Active:
		+local opportunities
		(logistic regression)

Age
Gender
Physical activity
  limitation
Education level
	Neighborhood features
	  (y/n): sidewalks, heavy
	  traffic, hills, street-
	  lights, unattended
	  dogs, enjoyable
	  scenery, frequently
	  see others exercising,
	  high levels of crime
	Neighborhood character
	  (3-point scale): rating
	  of neighborhood as
	  residential, mixed, or
	  commercial
	Neighborhood safety
	  (5-point scales): how
	  safe walking during
	  day
	Reported distance from
	  bikeway
	Reported steep hill on
	  way to bikeway
	Reported cross busy
	  street to access
	  bikeway
		Bikeway use:
		−reported distance (.65 times
		  as likely for every 0.25 in-
		  crease in distance)
		−busy street to cross (2 times
		  as likely if no street to cross)
		(logistic regression)

Age
Race
Education level
Geographic region
	Presence of (y/n): side-
	  walks, heavy traffic,
	  hills, streetlights, un-
	  attended dogs, enjoy-
		Not sedentary in rural women:
		+lack of scenery
		+frequency of seeing others
		  exercising

(continued)

TABLE 6-2 *(continued)* **Summary of Existing Research— Physical Activity Literature**

Study	Sampling	Survey	Physical Activity Variable
	BRFSS sampling plan	sectional survey	(based on moderate activity and vigorous activity)

NOTE: ANOVA = analysis of variance; BMI = body mass index; BRFSS = Behavioral Risk Factor Surveillance System; MAREPS = Methodology for the Analysis of the Rationality and Effectiveness of Prevention and Health Promotion Strategies; NHANES = National Health and Nutrition Examination Survey; SES = socioeconomic status.

[a] Sociodemographic and geographic variables only; many studies include other individual measures and social environment measures.

[b] Results of multivariate analyses reported when available.

[c] Included in Humpel et al. 2002.

Controls/ Confounders[a]	Built Environment Variables	Results[b]
	able scenery, frequently see others exercising, high levels of crime	
	Safe to walk or jog alone during the day (5-point scale)	
	Barriers (5-point scale): lack a safe place to exercise, poor weather	

REFERENCES

Abbreviations

BR&S	Belden, Russonello & Stewart
CDC	Centers for Disease Control and Prevention
EPA	U.S. Environmental Protection Agency
NCSA	National Center for Statistics and Analysis
NHTSA	National Highway Traffic Safety Administration
TRB	Transportation Research Board

Bagley, M. N., and P. L. Mokhtarian. 2002. The Impact of Residential Neighborhood Type on Travel Behavior: A Structural Equations Modeling Approach. *Annals of Regional Science*, Vol. 36, No. 2, pp. 279–297.

Ball, K., A. Bauman, E. Leslie, and N. Owen. 2001. Perceived Environmental Aesthetics and Convenience and Company Are Associated with Walking for Exercise Among Australian Adults. *Preventive Medicine*, Vol. 33, No. 5, pp. 434–440.

Berrigan, D., and R. P. Troiano. 2002. The Association Between Urban Form and Physical Activity in U.S. Adults. *American Journal of Preventive Medicine*, Vol. 23, No. 2S, pp. 74–79.

Black, C., A. Collins, and M. Snell. 2001. Encouraging Walking: The Case of Journey-to-School Trips in Compact Urban Areas. *Urban Studies*, Vol. 38, No. 7, pp. 1121–1141.

Boarnet, M. G. 2004. *The Built Environment and Physical Activity: Empirical Methods and Data Resources.* Prepared for the Committee on Physical Activity, Health, Transportation, and Land Use, July 18.

Boarnet, M. G., and R. Crane. 2001. *Travel by Design: The Influence of Urban Form on Travel.* Oxford University Press, New York.

Boarnet, M. G., K. Day, C. Anderson, T. McMillen, and M. Alfonzo. 2004. *Urban Form and Physical Activity: Insights from a Quasi-Experiment.* Presented at the Active Living Research Annual Conference, Del Mar, Calif., Jan. 30.

Boarnet, M. G., and S. Sarmiento. 1998. Can Land-Use Policy Really Affect Travel Behavior? A Study of the Link Between Non-Work Travel and Land-Use Characteristics. *Urban Studies*, Vol. 35, No. 7, June, pp. 1155–1169.

Booth, M. L., N. Owen, A. Bauman, O. Clavisi, and E. Leslie. 2000. Social-Cognitive and Perceived Environmental Influences Associated with Physical Activity in Older Australians. *Preventive Medicine*, Vol. 31, pp. 15–22.

Briss, P. A., S. Zaza, M. Pappaioanou, J. Fielding, L. Wright-De Agüero, B. I. Truman, D. P. Hopkins, P. Dolan Mullen, R. S. Thompson, S. H. Woolf, V. G. Carande-Kulis, L. Anderson, A. R. Hinman, D. V. McQueen, S. M. Teutsch, and J. R. Harris. 2000. Developing an Evidence-Based *Guide to Community Preventive Services*—Methods. *American Journal of Preventive Medicine*, Vol. 18, No. 1S, pp. 35–43.

Brownson, R. C., E. A. Baker, R. A. Housemann, L. K. Brennan, and S. J. Bacak. 2001. Environmental and Policy Determinants of Physical Activity in the United States. *American Journal of Public Health,* Vol. 91, No. 12, Dec.

Brownson, R. C., R. A. Housemann, D. R. Brown, J. Jackson-Thompson, A. C. King, B. R. Malone, and J. F. Sallis. 2000. Promoting Physical Activity in Rural Communities: Walking Trail Access, Use, and Effects. *American Journal of Preventive Medicine,* Vol. 18, No. 3, pp. 235–241.

BR&S. 2003. *Americans' Attitudes Toward Walking and Creating Better Walking Communities.* Washington, D.C., April.

Carande-Kulis, V. G., M. V. Maciosek, P. A. Briss, S. M. Teutsch, S. Zaza, B. I. Truman, M. L. Messonnier, M. Pappaioanou, J. R. Harris, and J. Fielding. 2000. Methods for Systematic Reviews of Economic Evaluations for the *Guide to Community Preventive Services. American Journal of Preventive Medicine,* Vol. 18, No. 1S, pp. 75–91.

CDC. 1999. Neighborhood Safety and the Prevalence of Physical Inactivity—Selected States, 1996. *Morbidity and Mortality Weekly Report,* Vol. 48, No. 7, pp. 143–146.

CDC. 2003. Prevalence of Physical Activity, Including Lifestyle Activities Among Adults—United States, 2000–2001. *Morbidity and Mortality Weekly Report,* Vol. 52, No. 32, pp. 764–769.

Cervero, R. 1996. Mixed Land-Uses and Commuting: Evidence from the American Housing Survey. *Transportation Research A,* Vol. 30, No. 5, pp. 361–377.

Cervero, R., and M. Duncan. 2002. *Residential Self Selection and Rail Commuting: A Nested Logit Analysis.* Working paper. University of California Transportation Center. www.uctc.net/papers/604.pdf.

Cervero, R., and M. Duncan. 2003. Walking, Bicycling, and Urban Landscapes: Evidence from the San Francisco Bay Area. *American Journal of Public Health,* Vol. 93, No. 9, pp. 1478–1483.

Cervero, R., and R. Gorham. 1995. Commuting in Transit Versus Automobile Neighborhoods. *Journal of the American Planning Association,* Vol. 61, No. 2, pp. 210–225.

Cervero, R., and K. Kockelman. 1997. Travel Demand and the 3 Ds: Density, Diversity, and Design. *Transportation Research D,* Vol. 2, No. 3, pp. 199–219.

Cervero, R., and C. Radisch. 1996. Travel Choices in Pedestrian Versus Automobile Oriented Neighborhoods. *Transport Policy,* Vol. 3, pp. 127–141.

Corless, J., and G. Ohland. 1999. *Caught in the Crosswalk.* www.transact.org/ca/caught99/ack.htm.

Craig, C. L., R. C. Brownson, S. E. Cragg, and A. L. Dunn. 2002. Exploring the Effect of the Environment on Physical Activity: A Study Examining Walking to Work. *American Journal of Preventive Medicine,* Vol. 23, No. 2S, pp. 36–43.

De Bourdeaudhuij, I., J. F. Sallis, and B. E. Saelens. 2003. Environmental Correlates of Physical Activity in a Sample of Belgian Adults. *American Journal of Health Promotion,* Vol. 18, No. 1, pp. 83–92.

Dellinger, A. M., and C. E. Staunton. 2002. Barriers to Children Walking and Cycling to School—United States, 1999. *Morbidity and Mortality Weekly Report,* Vol. 51, No. 32, Aug. 16, pp. 701–704.

Dorfman, R. A. 1997. Taking a Walk: No Longer Safe for Elders in Urban America and Asia. *Journal of Aging and Identity,* Vol. 2, No. 2, pp. 139–142.

Dunphy, R. T., and K. Fisher. 1996. Transportation, Congestion, and Density: New Insights. In *Transportation Research Record 1552,* TRB, National Research Council, Washington, D.C., pp. 89–96.

EPA. 2003. *Travel and Environmental Implications of School Siting.* EPA-231-R-03-004. Washington, D.C.

Evenson, K. R., O. L. Sarmiento, M. L. Macon, K. W. Tawney, and A. S. Ammerman. 2002. Environmental, Policy, and Cultural Factors Related to Physical Activity Among Latina Immigrants. *Women and Health,* Vol. 36, No. 2, pp. 43–57.

Ewing, R., P. Haliyur, and G. W. Page. 1994. Getting Around a Traditional City, a Suburban Planned Unit Development, and Everything in Between. In *Transportation Research Record 1466,* TRB, National Research Council, Washington, D.C., pp. 53–62.

Eyler, A. A., E. Baker, L. Cromer, A. C. King, R. C. Brownson, and R. J. Donatelle. 1998. Physical Activity and Minority Women: A Qualitative Study. *Health Education and Behavior,* Vol. 25, No. 5, pp. 640–652.

Eyler, A. A., D. Matson-Koffman, D. R. Young, S. Wilcox, J. Wilbur, J. L. Thompson, B. K. Sanderson, and K. R. Evenson. 2003. Quantitative Study of Correlates of Physical Activity in Women from Diverse Racial/Ethnic Groups: Women's Cardiovascular Health Network Project—Introduction and Methodology. *American Journal of Preventive Medicine,* Vol 25, No. 3Si, pp. 5–14.

Frank, L. D., and G. Pivo. 1994. Impacts of Mixed Use and Density on Utilization of Three Modes of Travel: Single-Occupant Vehicle, Transit, and Walking. In *Transportation Research Record 1466,* TRB, National Research Council, Washington, D.C., pp. 44–52.

Friedman, B., S. P. Gordon, and J. B. Peers. 1994. Effect of Neotraditional Neighborhood Design on Travel Characteristics. In *Transportation Research Record 1466,* TRB, National Research Council, Washington, D.C., pp. 63–70.

Giles-Corti, B., and R. J. Donovan. 2002a. Socioeconomic Status Differences in Recreational Physical Activity Levels and Real and Perceived Access to a Supportive Physical Environment. *Preventive Medicine,* Vol. 35, pp. 601–611.

Giles-Corti, B., and R. J. Donovan. 2002b. The Relative Influence of Individual, Social, and Environmental Determinants of Physical Activity. *Social Science and Medicine,* Vol. 54, pp. 1793–1812.

Giles-Corti, B., and R. J. Donovan. 2003. Relative Influences of Individual, Social Environmental, and Physical Environmental Correlates of Walking. *American Journal of Public Health,* Vol. 93, No. 9, pp. 1583–1589.

Greenwald, M. J., and M. G. Boarnet. 2001. Built Environment as Determinant of Walking Behavior: Analyzing Nonwork Pedestrian Travel in Portland, Oregon. In *Transportation Research Record: Journal of the Transportation Research Board, No. 1780,* TRB, National Research Council, Washington, D.C., pp. 33–42.

Handy, S. L. 1996a. Understanding the Link Between Urban Form and Nonwork Travel Behavior. *Journal of Planning Education and Research,* Vol. 15, No. 3, pp. 183–198.

Handy, S. L. 1996b. Urban Form and Pedestrian Choices: Study of Austin Neighborhoods. In *Transportation Research Record 1552,* TRB, National Research Council, Washington, D.C., pp. 135–144.

Handy, S. 2004. *Critical Assessment of the Literature on the Relationships Among Transportation, Land Use, and Physical Activity.* Department of Environmental Science and Policy, University of California, Davis. Prepared for the Committee on Physical Activity, Health, Transportation, and Land Use, July.

Handy, S. L., and K. J. Clifton. 2001. Local Shopping as a Strategy for Reducing Automobile Travel. *Transportation,* Vol. 28, No. 4, pp. 317–346.

Handy, S. L., K. J. Clifton, and J. Fisher. 1998. *The Effectiveness of Land Use Policies as a Strategy for Reducing Automobile Dependence: A Study of Austin Neighborhoods.* Center for Transportation Research, Southwest Region University Transportation Center, Austin, Tex.

Hanson, S., and M. Schwab. 1987. Accessibility and Intraurban Travel. *Environment and Planning A,* Vol. 19, pp. 735–748.

Hess, P. M., A. V. Moudon, M. C. Snyder, and K. Stanilov. 1999. Site Design and Pedestrian Travel. In *Transportation Research Record: Journal of the Transportation Research Board, No. 1674,* TRB, National Research Council, Washington, D.C., pp. 9–19.

Hoechner, C. M., L. K. Brennan, M. E. Elliott, S. L. Handy, and R. C. Brownson. In press. Perceived and Objective Environmental Measures and Physical Activity Among Urban Adults. *American Journal of Preventive Medicine.*

Hovell, M. F., J. F. Sallis, C. R. Hofstetter, V. M. Spry, P. Faucher, and C. J. Caspersen. 1989. Identifying Correlates of Walking for Exercise: An Epidemiologic Prerequisite for Physical Activity Promotion. *Preventive Medicine,* Vol. 18, No. 6, pp. 856–866.

Humpel, N., N. Owen., and E. Leslie. 2002. Environmental Factors Associated with Adults' Participation in Physical Activity: A Review. *American Journal of Preventive Medicine,* Vol. 22, No. 3, pp. 188–199.

Jacobsen, P. L. 2003. *Safety in Numbers: More Walkers and Bicyclists, Safer Walking and Biking.* Cited in University of California–Berkeley Traffic Safety Center Issue of Safety, Physical Activity, and the Built Environment, Vol. 2, No. 1, Spring 2004.

Jacobsen, P. L., C. Anderson, D. Winn, J. Moffat, P. Agran, and S. Sarkar. 2000. Child Pedestrian Injuries on Residential Streets: Implications for Traffic Engineering. *Institute of Transportation Engineering Journal on the Web,* Feb., pp. 71–75.

Kahn, E. B., L. T. Ramsey, R. C. Brownson, G. W. Heath, E. H. Howze, K. E. Powell, E. J. Stone, M. W. Rajab, and P. Corso. 2002. The Effectiveness of Interventions to Increase Physical Activity: A Systematic Review. *American Journal of Preventive Medicine*, Vol. 22, No. 4S, pp. 73–107.

Kerr, N. A., M. M. Yore, S. A. Ham, and W. H. Dietz. 2004. Increasing Stair Use in a Worksite Through Environmental Changes. *American Journal of Health Promotion*, Vol. 18, No. 4, March–April, pp. 312–315.

King, A. C., C. Castro, S. Wilcox, A. A. Eyler, J. F. Sallis, and R. C. Brownson. 2000. Personal and Environmental Factors Associated with Physical Inactivity Among Different Racial-Ethnic Groups of U.S. Middle-Aged and Older-Aged Women. *Health Psychology*, Vol. 19, No. 4, pp. 354–364.

Kitamura, R., P. L. Mokhtarian, and L. Laidet. 1997. A Micro-Analysis of Land Use and Travel in Five Neighborhoods in the San Francisco Bay Area. *Transportation*, Vol. 24, No. 2, pp. 125–158.

Klinenberg, E. 2002. *Heat Wave: A Social Autopsy of Disaster in Chicago*. University of Chicago Press, Chicago, Ill.

Kockelman, K. M. 1997. Travel Behavior as Function of Accessibility, Land Use Mixing, and Land Use Balance: Evidence from San Francisco Bay Area. In *Transportation Research Record 1607*, TRB, National Research Council, Washington, D.C., pp. 116–125.

Krizek, K. J. 2000. Pretest-Posttest Strategy for Researching Neighborhood-Scale Urban Form and Travel Behavior. In *Transportation Research Record: Journal of the Transportation Research Board, No. 1722*, TRB, National Research Council, Washington, D.C., pp. 48–55.

Krizek, K. J. 2003. Residential Relocation and Changes in Urban Travel: Does Neighborhood-Scale Urban Form Matter? *Journal of the American Planning Association*, Vol. 69, No. 3, Summer, pp. 265–279.

Levine, N., K. Kim, and L. Nitz. 1994. Traffic Safety and Land Use: A Spatial Analysis of Honolulu Motor Vehicle Accidents. Presented at the 1994 ACSP Conference, Phoenix, Ariz.

Los Angeles Times. 1999. Walk to School Hazardous for Santa Ana Kids. May 27.

Loukaitou-Sideris, A. 2004. *Transportation, Land Use, and Physical Activity: Safety and Security Considerations*. Prepared for the Committee on Physical Activity, Health, Transportation, and Land Use, June.

MacDougall, C., R. Cooke, N. Owen, K. Willson, and A. Bauman. 1997. Relating Physical Activity to Health Status, Social Connections and Community Facilities. *Australian and New Zealand Journal of Public Health*, Vol. 21, No. 6, pp. 631–637.

McCormack, E., G. S. Rutherford, and M. G. Wilkinson. 2001. Travel Impacts of Mixed Land Use Neighborhoods in Seattle, Washington. In *Transportation Research Record:*

Journal of the Transportation Research Board, No. 1780, TRB, National Research Council, Washington, D.C., pp. 25–32.

McNally, M. G., and A. Kulkarni. 1997. Assessment of Influence of Land Use–Transportation System on Travel Behavior. In *Transportation Research Record 1607*, TRB, National Research Council, Washington, D.C., pp. 105–115.

Messenger, T., and R. Ewing. 1996. Transit-Oriented Development in the Sun Belt. In *Transportation Research Record 1552*, TRB, National Research Council, Washington, D.C., pp. 145–153.

Molnar, B. E., S. L. Gortmaker, F. C. Bull, and S. L. Buka. 2004. Unsafe to Play? Neighborhood Disorder and Lack of Safety Predict Reduced Physical Activity Among Urban Children and Adolescents. *American Journal of Health Promotion*, Vol. 18, No. 5, pp. 378–386.

Moudon, A. V., P. M. Hess, M. C. Snyder, and K. Stanilov. 1997. Effect of Site Design on Pedestrian Travel in Mixed-Use, Medium-Density Environments. In *Transportation Research Record 1578*, TRB, National Research Council, Washington, D.C., pp. 48–55.

NCSA. 2003a. *Traffic Safety Facts 2003: Pedalcyclists.* DOT-HS-809-768. U.S. Department of Transportation. www-nrd.nhtsa.dot.gov/pdf/nrd-30/NCSA/TSF2003/809768.pdf. Accessed Nov. 23, 2004.

NCSA. 2003b. *Traffic Safety Facts 2003: Pedestrians.* DOT-HS-809-769. U.S. Department of Transportation. www-nrd.nhtsa.dot.gov/pdf/nrd-30/NCSA/TSF2003/809769.pdf. Accessed Nov. 23, 2004.

Parks, S. E., R. A. Housemann, and R. C. Brownson. 2003. Differential Correlates of Physical Activity in Urban and Rural Adults of Various Socioeconomic Backgrounds in the United States. *Journal of Epidemiology and Community Health*, Vol. 57, No. 1, pp. 29–35.

Parsons Brinckerhoff Quade & Douglas. 1993. *The Pedestrian Environment.* 1000 Friends of Oregon, Portland.

Powell, K. E., L. M. Martin, and P. P. Chowdhury. 2003. Places to Walk: Convenience and Regular Physical Activity. *American Journal of Public Health*, Vol. 93, No. 9, pp. 1519–1521.

Pushkarev, B. S., and J. M. Zupan. 1977. *Public Transportation and Land Use Policy.* Indiana University Press, Bloomington.

Rodriguez, D. A., A. J. Khattak, and K. Evenson. 2005. Can Neighborhood Design Encourage Walking and Bicycling? Physical Activity in New Urbanist and Conventional Suburban Communities. Presented at 84th Annual Meeting of the Transportation Research Board.

Ross, C. E. 2000. Walking, Exercising, and Smoking: Does Neighborhood Matter? *Social Science and Medicine*, Vol. 51, No. 2, pp. 265–274.

Rutten, A., T. Abel, L. Kannas, T. von Lengerke, G. Luschen, J. A. Diaz, J. Vinck, and J. van der Zee. 2001. Self Reported Physical Activity, Public Health, and Perceived Environment: Results from a Comparative European Study. *Journal of Epidemiology and Community Health,* Vol. 55, No. 2, pp. 139–146.

Saelens, B. E., J. F. Sallis, and L. D. Frank. 2003. Environmental Correlates of Walking and Cycling: Findings from the Transportation, Urban Design, and Planning Literatures. *Annals of Behavioral Medicine,* Vol. 25, No. 2, pp. 80–91.

Saelens, B. E., J. F. Sallis, J. B. Black, and D. Chen. 2003. Neighborhood-Based Differences in Physical Activity: An Environment Scale Evaluation. *American Journal of Public Health,* Vol. 93, No. 9, pp. 1552–1558.

Sallis, J. F., A. Bauman, and M. Pratt. 1998. Environmental and Policy Interventions to Promote Physical Activity. *American Journal of Preventive Medicine,* Vol. 15, No. 4, pp. 379–397.

Sallis, J. F., M. F. Hovell, and C. R. Hofstetter. 1992. Predictors of Adoption and Maintenance of Vigorous Physical Activity in Men and Women. *Preventive Medicine,* Vol. 21, No. 2, pp. 237–251.

Sallis, J. F., M. F. Hovell, C. R. Hofstetter, J. P. Elder, M. Hackley, C. J. Caspersen, and K. E. Powell. 1990. Distance Between Homes and Exercise Facilities Related to Frequency of Exercise Among San Diego Residents. *Public Health Reports,* Vol. 105, No. 2, pp. 179–185.

Sallis, J. F., M. F. Hovell, C. R. Hofstetter, P. Faucher, J. P. Elder, J. Blanchard, C. J. Caspersen, K. E. Powell, and G. M. Christenson. 1989. A Multivariate Study of Determinants of Vigorous Exercise in a Community Sample. *Preventive Medicine,* Vol. 18, No. 1, pp. 20–34.

Sallis, J. F., M. F. Johnson, K. J. Calfas, S. Caparosa, and J. F. Nichols. 1997. Assessing Perceived Physical Environmental Variables That May Influence Physical Activity. *Research Quarterly for Exercise and Sport,* Vol. 68, No. 4, pp. 345–351.

Sallis, J. F., T. L. McKenzie, J. P. Elder, S. L. Broyles, and P. R. Nader. 1997. Factors Parents Use in Selecting Play Spaces for Young Children. *Archives of Pediatrics and Adolescent Medicine,* Vol. 151, pp. 414–417.

Schimek, P. 1996. Household Motor Vehicle Ownership and Use: How Much Does Residential Density Matter? In *Transportation Research Record 1552,* TRB, National Research Council, Washington, D.C., pp. 120–125.

Schwanen, T., and P. Mokhtarian. 2004. What Affects Commute Mode Choice: Neighborhood Physical Structure or Preferences Toward Neighborhoods? *Journal of Transport Geography,* forthcoming.

Seefeldt, V., R. M. Malina, and M. A. Clark. 2002. Factors Affecting Levels of Physical Activity in Adults (Review). *Sports Medicine,* Vol. 32, No. 3, pp. 143–168.

Sharpe, P. A., M. L. Granner, B. Hutto, and B. E. Ainsworth. 2004. Association of Environmental Factors to Meeting Physical Activity Recommendations in Two South Carolina Counties. *American Journal of Health Promotion,* Vol. 18, No. 3, Jan.–Feb., pp. 251–258.

Sharples, P. M., A. Storey, A. Aynsley-Green, and J. A. Eyre. 1990. Causes of Fatal Childhood Accidents Involving Head Injury in Northern Region, 1979–1986. *British Medical Journal,* Vol. 301, pp. 1193–1197.

Shaw, S. M., A. Bonen, and J. F. McCabe. 1991. Do More Constraints Mean Less Leisure? Examining the Relationship Between Constraints and Participation. *Journal of Leisure Research,* Vol. 23, No. 4, pp. 286–300.

Stahl, T., A. Rutten, D. Nutbeam, A. Bauman, L. Kannas, T. Abel, G. Luschen, D. J. Rodriquez, J. Vinck, and J. van der Zee. 2001. The Importance of the Social Environment for Physically Active Lifestyle—Results from an International Study. *Social Science and Medicine,* Vol. 52, No. 1, pp. 1–10.

Thompson, J. L., P. Allen, L. Cunningham-Sabo, D. Yazzie, M. Curtis, and S. M. Davis. 2002. Environmental, Policy and Cultural Factors Related to Physical Activity in Sedentary American Indian Women. *Women and Health,* Vol. 36, No. 2, pp. 59–74.

TRB. 1995. *Special Report 245: Expanding Metropolitan Highways: Implications for Air Quality and Energy Use.* National Research Council, Washington, D.C.

TRB. 2001. *Special Report 257: Making Transit Work: Insight from Western Europe, Canada, and the United States.* National Research Council, Washington, D.C.

TRB. 2002. *Special Report 269: The Relative Risks of School Travel: A National Perspective and Guidance for Local Community Risk Assessment.* National Research Council, Washington, D.C.

Troped, P. J., R. P. Saunders, R. R. Pate, B. Reininger, J. R. Ureda, and S. J. Thompson. 2001. Associations Between Self-Reported and Objective Physical Environmental Factors and Use of a Community Rail-Trail. *Preventive Medicine,* Vol. 32, No. 2, pp. 191–200.

Valentine, G., and J. H. McKendrick. 1997. Children Outdoor Play: Exploring Parental Concerns About Children's Safety and the Changing Nature of Childhood. *Geoforum,* Vol. 28, pp. 219–235.

Walgren, S. 1998. *Using Geographic Information Systems (GIS) to Analyze Pedestrian Accidents.* Transportation Department, City of Seattle, Wash. www.cityofseattle.net/td/ite.asp.

Wegmann, F. J., and T. Y. Jang. 1998. Trip Linkage Patterns for Workers. *Journal of Transportation Engineering,* May–June, pp. 264–270.

Wilbur, J., P. Chandler, B. Dancy, J. Choi, and D. Plonczynski. 2002. Environmental, Policy, and Cultural Factors Related to Physical Activity in Urban, African-American Women. *Women and Health,* Vol. 36, No. 2, pp. 17–28.

Wilcox, S., C. Castro, A. C. King, R. Housemann, and R. C. Brownson. 2000. Determinants of Leisure Time Physical Activity in Rural Compared with Urban Older and Ethnically Diverse Women in the United States. *Journal of Epidemiology and Community Health,* Vol. 54, No. 9, pp. 667–672.

Young, D. R., X. He, J. Harris, and I. Mabry. 2002. Environmental, Policy, and Cultural Factors Related to Physical Activity in Well-Educated Urban African-American Women. *Women and Health,* Vol. 36, No. 2, pp. 29–41.

Zimring, C., A. Joseph, G. L. Nicoll, and S. Tsepas. 2004. Influences of Building Design and Site Design on Physical Activity: Research and Intervention Opportunities. *American Journal of Preventive Medicine* (in review).

7

Future Directions

In this chapter, the committee presents its detailed consensus findings, conclusions, and recommendations. First, however, it should be emphasized that research on the relationship between the built environment and physical activity is at a pivotal stage. A growing body of empirical evidence, primarily from cross-sectional studies reviewed in Chapter 6, suggests an association between the built environment and physical activity levels. The science, however, is not sufficiently advanced to support causal connections or identify with certainty those characteristics of the built environment most closely associated with physical activity behavior. Thus, the committee is unable to provide specific policy guidance, although it offers several recommendations for strengthening theory, research, and data that should provide a firmer basis for future policy making and intervention.

The committee believes that the importance of physical activity to health warrants a strong and continuing research effort to further understand the relationship between the built environment and physical activity. If the field is to move forward, however, different kinds of collaboration and research are needed. First, a more interdisciplinary approach to research would help bring together the needed expertise of the public health, physical activity, urban planning, and transportation communities, among others. The committee found that the interdisciplinary character of its own membership greatly facilitated its understanding of the issues. Second, researchers should broaden their areas of inquiry to address the knowledge gaps identified in Chapter 6. Third, additional funding is needed to support difficult-to-finance multiyear longitudinal studies, rapid-response capability to evaluate natural experiments as they arise, and extensions of national databases if important causal connections are to be researched.[1] Among the committee's key recommendations is support for a collaborative effort by the leadership of the Department of Health and Human Services and the Department of Transportation through an interagency working group to help develop and fund an appropriate research agenda for this purpose.

Finally, the committee wishes to emphasize that, as noted in Chapter 6, modifications to the built environment alone are unlikely to solve the public health problem of insufficient physical activity. Increasing populationwide levels of physical activity will require a range of approaches. Complementary strategies addressing the individual and social as well as the environmental determinants of physical activity behavior need to be the subject of future research and interventions. Such complementary strategies need to encompass leisure-time, home-based, transport, and occupation-based physical activity, given that a combination of physical activities in a variety of settings and locations can provide individuals with a feasible way to reach the goal of at least 30 minutes per day of moderate physical activity.[2] The fact that this 30 minutes can be accumulated in segments of at least 10 minutes (see Chapter 2) means that all the activity need not be accrued in leisure time, at home, in transport, or at work, but can be spread across a range of locations where individuals spend their time.

---

[1] A review of research in progress under the sponsorship of the Active Living Research Program of the Robert Wood Johnson Foundation found few longitudinal studies in the pipeline. While it is committed to the concept of longitudinal studies, the foundation does not have the resources to support large-scale, multiyear longitudinal studies.

[2] Practically speaking, reaching the daily guideline of 30 minutes may require additional time both before and after the activity (e.g., changing clothes, showering, travel to and from a gym or recreation area). The amount of additional time, however, depends on the location and type of activity. Three 10-minute walks per day inserted into routine daily activities—such as a 10-minute walk before breakfast, at lunchtime, and after dinner—require no more than a total of 30 minutes per day.

FINDINGS

Physical activity levels have declined sharply over the past half-century because of reduced physical demands of work, household management, and travel, together with increased sedentary uses of free time. Labor-saving technological innovations have brought comfort, convenience, and time for more leisure activities. They have resulted as well in more sedentary lifestyles with adverse health effects for many Americans. Changes in land use and travel may also have contributed to the decline in physical activity levels. For example, the steady dispersion of both population and employment to low-density suburban locations has increased reliance on the private vehicle as the dominant and most convenient travel mode. Rebuilding physical activity into the daily routine is a public health priority, but the specific contribution that the built environment could make is not well understood.

The built environment can facilitate or constrain physical activity. The built environment can be structured in ways that give people more or fewer opportunities and choices to be physically active. The characteristics of the built environment that facilitate or constrain physical activity may differ depending on the purpose of the activity. For example, ready access to parks and trails may facilitate walking for exercise; sidewalks and mixed-use development are likely to be more important to encourage walking for local shopping and other utilitarian purposes. The built environment can be changed in ways that increase opportunities for and reduce barriers to physical activity. The paradigm of the Robert Wood Johnson Foundation's "active living" concept, for example, is to make opportunities for physical activity so pervasive that such activity is integrated into daily routines.

The relationship between the built environment and physical activity is complex and operates through many mediating factors, such as sociodemographic characteristics, personal and cultural variables, safety and security, and time allocation. Whether an individual is physically active is determined largely by his or her capacity, propensity, and willingness to make time for physical activity. For example, while public health surveys have found that on average physical activity levels decline with age, many senior citizens remain physically active. Individual behavior is also influenced by the social and physical environment (see Figure 1-1 in Chapter 1). For example, the social disorder and deteriorated physical condition of poor inner-city neighborhoods deter physical activity for many residents. These neighborhoods have some of the physical characteristics thought to be conducive to walking and nonmotorized transport—sidewalks, multiple destinations within close proximity, and mixed land uses—and indeed, low-income urban populations report high levels of walking for utilitarian trips. However, they also report low levels of discretionary physical activity. Crime-ridden streets, littered sidewalks, and poorly maintained environments discourage outdoor physical activity other than necessary trips. Time is another mediating factor, cited by many as a reason for not being more physically active. For some (e.g., single parents, those holding two jobs), making time for physical activity is difficult. For others, particularly those who spend large amounts of leisure time on such sedentary pursuits as watching television, sedentary behavior may reflect the low priority given to physical activity. Time constraints often dominate the choice of travel mode, particularly for destination-oriented trips such as commuting and shopping, and influence destination and activity choices. In general, the role of time has not been well accounted for in examining the relationship between the built environment and physical activity.

The available empirical evidence shows an association between the built environment and physical activity. However, few studies capable of demonstrating a causal relationship have been conducted, and evidence supporting such a relationship is currently sparse. In addition, the characteristics of the built environment most closely associated with physical activity remain to be determined. Preliminary research does provide some evidence suggesting that such factors as access and safety and security are important for some forms of physical activity, such as walking and cycling, and for some population groups. However, the findings are not definitive because it is not known whether these characteristics affect a person's overall level of physical activity or just his or her amount of outdoor walking and cycling. Furthermore, the literature has not established the degree of impact of the built environment and its various characteristics on physical activity levels; the variance by location (e.g., inner city, inner suburb, outer suburb) and population subgroup (e.g., children, the elderly, the disadvantaged); or the importance to total physical activity levels, the primary variable of interest from a public health perspective.

Weaknesses of the current literature include the lack of a sound theoretical framework, inadequate research designs, and incomplete data. The current state of knowledge in this area is limited in part by the lack of a sound theoretical framework to guide empirical work and inadequate research designs. As noted, most of the studies conducted to date have been cross-sectional. Longitudinal study designs using time-series data are also needed to investigate causal relationships between the built environment and physical activity. Studies that distinguish carefully between personal attitudes and choices and external influences on observed behavior are needed to determine how much an observed association between the built environment and physical activity—for example, in an activity-friendly neighborhood—reflects the physical characteristics of the neighborhood versus the lifestyle preferences of those who choose to live there. Appropriate measures of the built environment are still being developed, and efforts to link such measures to travel and health databases are at an early stage. For example, none of the national public health surveys on physical activity report its location or include such activity within buildings, although physical activity often takes place in workplaces, homes, and schools. Travel surveys are typically focused on purposeful travel and ignore physical activity for exercise or recreation.[3] Another issue is the appropriate scale of the built environment to which physical activity data should be linked and the relevant environmental characteristics that should be included at each

---

[3] The distinction between physical activity for exercise and for transportation, however, is not always clear. For example, an individual could walk to neighborhood shopping both for exercise and to run errands.

scale. For example, design features that may encourage walking within buildings or at building sites are likely to differ from those that may encourage physical activity in a neighborhood or the larger community.

The built environment in place today has been shaped by long-standing policies and the practices of many decision makers (e.g., policy makers, elected officials, planners, developers, traffic engineers). Many existing development patterns have resulted from zoning and land use ordinances, design guidelines and funding criteria for transportation infrastructure focused primarily on motorized transportation, values and preferences of home owners and home buyers (e.g., suburban lifestyles, single-family housing), and racial and economic concentration of the poor and disinvestment in their neighborhoods. At the same time, the built environment is constantly changing as homes are renovated and new residences, developments, and office complexes are constructed.

CONCLUSIONS

Regular physical activity is important for health, and inadequate physical activity is a major, largely preventable public health problem.

The committee concurs with the strong and well-established scientific evidence linking physical activity to health outcomes and supporting reversal of the decline in overall physical activity levels as a public health priority. The connection between regular physical activity and health, although not the primary focus of this study, has clearly motivated interest in examining the built environment as a potential point of intervention to encourage more active behavior.

Built environments that facilitate more active lifestyles and reduce barriers to physical activity are desirable because of the positive relationship between physical activity and health.

Achieving this goal is challenging in a highly technological society with a built environment that is already in place and often expensive to change. Nevertheless, even small increases in physical activity levels can have important health and economic benefits. Moreover, the built environment is constantly being renovated and rebuilt and new developments are being constructed; these changes provide opportunities to incorporate more activity-conducive environments. In the committee's judgment, such changes would be desirable even in the absence of the goal of increasing physical activity because of their positive social effects on neighborhood safety, sense of community, and quality of life.

Continuing modifications to the built environment provide opportunities, over time, to institute policies and practices that support the provision of more activity-conducive environments.

The long-term decline in physical activity among the U.S. population has been the cumulative result of many changes; thus there are many opportunities for intervention. However, some interventions will be easier to effect than others. For example, formidable hurdles would have to be overcome to substantially modify long-standing policies, such as the current system of zoning regulations and land use controls that reflects the preferences of many suburban home owners and buyers, to allow greater density of development and more mixed land uses. Similarly, many barriers persist to ending concentrations of minority populations and underinvestment in poor neighborhoods and the accompanying social and economic isolation of the poor. More flexible and targeted approaches—context-sensitive design, special overlay districts, traffic calming measures, community policing—have a better chance of gaining support. Construction of new buildings and developments offers promising opportunities for creating more activity-friendly environments. A wider range of such environments should become available as more neotraditional communities prove financially successful and employers embrace more walking-friendly office complexes to encourage healthier workforces.

Opportunities to increase physical activity levels exist in many settings—at home, at work, at school, in travel, and in leisure. The built environment has the potential to influence physical activity in each of these settings.

Each setting is characterized by different environmental opportunities and constraints that could affect physical activity levels. In some neighborhoods, for example, residents walk for utilitarian purposes. Keeping these neighborhoods safe and providing desirable destinations should help reinforce and perhaps enhance this behavior. In other neighborhoods, walking for utilitarian purposes is limited. In these settings, recreational walking and cycling may offer the greatest potential for increasing physical activity in the daily routine. Trend data from national public health surveys suggest that in fact leisure-time physical activity has increased slightly over the past decade, and the literature reveals that many characteristics of the built environment at the neighborhood level are significantly correlated with leisure-time physical activity and exercise. Of course, individuals can also obtain their daily physical activity by exercising at home. Most Americans spend the majority of their day at home, at work, and at school, and these are important but understudied locations for physical activity, particularly in view of the guidelines, which suggest that the daily 30-minute minimum of moderate physical activity can be accumulated in many locations and in small (10-minute) time increments.

Many opportunities and potential policies exist for changing the built environment in ways that are more conducive to physical activity, but the available evidence is not sufficient to identify which specific changes would have the most impact on physical activity levels and health outcomes.

Research has not yet identified causal relationships to a point that would enable the committee to provide guidance about cost-beneficial investments or state unequivocally that certain changes to the built environment would lead to more physical activity or be the most efficient ways of increasing such activity. Effective policies to this end are likely to differ for different population groups (e.g., children, youths, the elderly, the disadvantaged), for different purposes of physical activity (e.g., transportation, exercise), and in different contexts (e.g., inner city, inner suburb, outer suburb, rural). For example, much recent research has focused appropriately on physical activity at the neighborhood level, where many opportunities exist for walking and cycling for recreation or errands. However, home and work can also be locations for physical activity, as can travel itself between home and work or other destinations.

RECOMMENDATIONS

Given the current state of knowledge and the importance of physical activity for health, the committee urges a continuing and well-supported research effort in this area, which Congress should include in its authorization of research funding for health, physical activity, transportation, planning, and other related areas.

Priorities for this research include the following:

- *Interdisciplinary approaches and international collaboration* bringing together the expertise of the public health, physical activity, urban planning, and transportation research communities, among others, both in the United States and abroad.
- *More complete conceptual models* that provide the basis for formulating testable hypotheses, suggesting the variables and relationships for analysis, and interpreting the results.
- *Better research designs,* particularly longitudinal studies that can begin to address causality issues, as well as designs that control more adequately for self-selection bias.
- *More detailed examination and matching of specific characteristics of the built environment with different types of physical activity* to assess the strength of the relationship and the proportion of affected population subgroups. All types of physical activity

should be included because there may be substitution among different types. The goal from a public health perspective is an increase in total physical activity levels.

National public health and travel surveys should be expanded to provide more detailed information about the locations of physical activity and travel, which is fundamental to understanding the link between the built environment and physical activity in all potential contexts.

Geocoding the data on physical activity and health collected in large surveys, such as the Behavioral Risk Factor Surveillance System, the National Health and Nutrition Examination Survey, and the National Health Interview Survey, could help link these rich data sets with information on the built environment and the specific locations where physical activity is occurring. Similarly, travel surveys, such as the National Household Travel Survey, as well as regional travel surveys, should be geocoded to provide more fine-grained geographic detail so researchers can link these surveys and diary data with characteristics of the built environment. In addition, data that reflect a more comprehensive picture of physical activity should be provided. For the public health databases, this means capturing more than leisure-time physical activity; for the travel databases, a more complete accounting should be provided of walking and other forms of nonmotorized travel. More reliable and valid measures of the built environment, both objective and subjective, are also needed. Technologies are available to help verify the accuracy of self-reported data automatically and objectively. Ideally, both self-reported and objectively measured data should be collected. Self-reported data provide qualitative insights, such as trip purpose, that cannot be determined through technical measurement, while objective measures reduce the risks of respondent bias and provide a cross-check of survey responses. Finally, a new database—the Bureau of Labor Statistics' American Time Use Survey—provides an opportunity to track detailed types and durations of respondent activities in many locations. With the collection of extensive demographic and socioeconomic data on the respondents, the database offers researchers a more comprehensive picture of activities and time-use trade-offs by various subgroups of the population than has previously been available. Because the survey is new, opportunities exist to add questions related specifically to physical activity levels.

When changes are made to the built environment—whether retrofitting existing environments or constructing new developments or communities—researchers should view such natural experiments as "demonstration" projects and analyze their impacts on physical activity.

Numerous such opportunities exist, ranging from the construction of new, neotraditional developments to projects of the Active Living by Design Program of the Robert Wood Johnson Foundation.[4] To take advantage of these natural experiments, baseline data must be collected. A "rapid-response" capability is needed so that timely funding can be made available to gather the appropriate data when opportunities arise. This might mean gathering data in both treatment and comparison communities prior to an intervention to provide before and after data for assessing impacts.

Leadership of the Department of Health and Human Services and the Department of Transportation should work collaboratively through an interagency working group to shape an appropriate research agenda and develop a specific recommendation to Congress for a program of research with a defined mission and recommended budget.

An interagency approach is needed because the necessary research does not fall within the purview of any one agency. The committee recognizes that funding for research is currently being provided by the Robert Wood Johnson Foundation and encourages its continuation. Additional funding is needed to enhance research and data

---

[4] This program funds projects to develop, implement, and evaluate approaches that support physical activity and promote active living. Partnerships involving local, state, and regional public and nonprofit organizations are eligible and receive grants of up to $200,000 over 5 years.

collection in several areas and provide a more solid foundation for policy making. An interagency initiative is likely to encourage a more interdisciplinary approach to the problem.

Federally supported research funding should be targeted to high-payoff but difficult-to-finance multiyear projects and enhanced data collection.

The highest priorities, in the committee's judgment, include funding for multiyear longitudinal studies, a rapid-response capability to take advantage of natural experiments as they arise, and support for recommended additions to national databases. The federal government should supplement funding provided by foundations to ensure that this high-payoff research is conducted. The new National Institutes of Health initiative on obesity and the built environment is one possible funding source.[5]

The committee encourages the study of a combined strategy of social marketing and changes to the built environment as interventions to increase physical activity.[6]

The research should be designed to study these approaches both separately and in combination so that the influence of individual factors can be evaluated. To be effective, social marketing campaigns should be tailored to different population subgroups with relatively homogeneous characteristics and linked with other interventions involving the built environment for evaluation. For example, a social marketing campaign targeted to low-income, minority popula-

---

[5] This new program, sponsored by the National Institutes of Health, provides grants to study the impact of the built environment on being overweight and obese. For Fiscal Year 2005, $5 million is committed to support studies that will (*a*) further understanding of the role of the built environment in causing or exacerbating obesity and related comorbidities and (*b*) develop, implement, and evaluate prevention and intervention strategies designed to influence characteristics of the built environment so as to reduce the prevalence of being overweight and obese. Grantees must be interdisciplinary partners from the public health and transportation fields.

[6] Social marketing is the application of commercial marketing techniques to the analysis, planning, execution, and evaluation of programs designed to influence the voluntary behavior of target audiences so as to improve their personal welfare and that of their society.

tions could be combined with a community policing effort to create safe havens for walking and studied for the effect on increasing physical activity levels in these communities. This targeted approach should prove more effective than mass messages about the benefits of being physically active. Possible audiences include but are not limited to (*a*) subgroups of the population segmented by gender, age, income, and race; (*b*) public and private officials responsible for community design, development, safety, and public health (e.g., elected officials, planners and planning boards, parks departments, local police, local public health officials, developers); (*c*) transportation infrastructure planners and providers (e.g., metropolitan planning organizations, traffic engineers and consultants), and (*d*) private employers responsible for workplace design and employee information programs and incentives.

Universities should develop interdisciplinary education programs to train professionals in conducting the recommended research and prepare practitioners with appropriate skills at the intersection of physical activity, public health, transportation, and urban planning.

Ideally, new interdisciplinary programs should be developed with a core curriculum that brings together the public health, physical activity, transportation, and urban planning fields in a focused program on the built environment and physical activity. At a minimum, existing programs in public health, transportation, and urban planning should be expanded to provide courses related to physical activity, the built environment, and public health. Similarly, practitioners in the field—local public health workers, physical activity specialists, traffic engineers, and local urban planners—could benefit from supplemental training in these areas.

Those responsible for modifications or additions to the built environment should facilitate access to, enhance the attractiveness of, and ensure the safety and security of places where people can be physically active.

Even though causal connections between the built environment and physical activity levels have not been demonstrated in the literature to date, the available evidence suggests that the built environment can play a facilitating role by providing places and inducements for people to be physically active. Local planning officials, as well as those responsible for the design and construction of residences, developments, and supporting transportation infrastructure, should be encouraged to provide more activity-friendly environments.

APPENDIX A

COMMISSIONED PAPERS AND AUTHORS

The Built Environment and Physical Activity: Empirical Methods and Data Resources. Marlon G. Boarnet, Department of Urban and Regional Planning, University of California, Irvine, July 18, 2004.

Consumer Preferences and Social Marketing Approaches to Physical Activity Behavior and Transportation and Land Use Choices. Susan D. Kirby, Kirby Marketing Solutions, Inc., and Marla Hollander, Leadership for Active Living, San Diego State University, April 19, 2004.

Critical Assessment of the Literature on the Relationships Among Transportation, Land Use, and Physical Activity. Susan Handy, Department of Environmental Science and Policy, University of California, Davis, July 2004.

Institutional and Regulatory Factors Related to Nonmotorized Travel and Walkable Communities. Michael D. Meyer and Eric Dumbaugh, School of Civil and Environmental Engineering, Georgia Institute of Technology, July 5, 2004.

Patterns and Trends in Physical Activity, Occupation, Transportation, Land Use, and Sedentary Behaviors. Ross C. Brownson and Tegan K. Boehmer, School of Public Health, Saint Louis University, June 25, 2004.

Promoting Interdisciplinary Curricula and Training in Transportation, Land Use, Physical Activity, and Health. Elliott D. Sclar, Urban Planning and Public Affairs, Columbia University; Mary E. Northridge and Emily M. Karpel, Mailman School of Public Health, Columbia University, June 29, 2004.

Transportation, Land Use, and Physical Activity: Safety and Security Concerns. Anastasia Loukaitou-Sideris, School of Public Policy and Research, University of California, Los Angeles, June 2004.

NOTE: The commissioned papers are available at
trb.org/downloads/sr282papers/sr282paperstoc.pdf.

WORKSHOP AGENDA
AND PARTICIPANTS

The National Academies
Transportation Research Board
Institute of Medicine

Workshop on Physical Activity, Health, Transportation, and Land Use

The George and Martha Mitchell Conference Center
at The Keck Center of the National Academies,
500 Fifth Street, NW, Washington, D.C.
Thursday, December 11, 2003

AGENDA

8:30–8:35 a.m.	**Welcome and Overview** Susan Hanson, Committee Chair
8:35–10:15 a.m.	**Panel 1: Overview of the Trends and Evidence Available on the Relationships Among Physical Activity, Transportation, and Land Use** Paper moderators (Genevieve Giuliano and Kenneth Powell, respectively)
8:35–9:25 a.m.	**A Half-Century of Change: Trends in Population, Land Use, Transportation, and Physical Activity**

235

Paper authors—Ross Brownson and Tegan Boehmer, School of Public Health, St. Louis University

Commentator—Joseph L. Schofer, Robert R. McCormick School of Engineering and Applied Science, Northwestern University

9:25–10:15 a.m. **Assessment of the Literature on the Relationships Among Physical Activity, Transportation, and Land Use**
Paper author—Susan L. Handy, Department of Environmental Science and Policy, University of California at Davis

Commentator—Brian D. Taylor, School of Public Policy and Social Research, University of California at Los Angeles

10:15–10:30 a.m. Break

10:30 a.m.– **Panel 2: Data and Fostering Behavior**
12:10 p.m. **Change to Increase Physical Activity Through Transportation and Land Use Choices**
Paper moderators (Jane C. Stutts and Bobbie A. Berkowitz, respectively)

10:30– **Current and Future Data and**
11:20 a.m. **Data Sources for Evaluating These Relationships**
Paper author—Marlon G. Boarnet, Department of Planning, Policy, and Design, University of California at Irvine

Commentator—Loretta DiPietro, Department of Environmental Health, Yale School of Public Health

11:20 a.m.– **Consumer Preferences, Marketing,**
12:10 p.m **and Social Marketing Approaches**

Paper authors—Susan D. Kirby, Kirby Marketing Solutions, Inc., and Marla Hollander, Leadership for Active Living, San Diego State University

Commentator—Ed Maibach, National Cancer Institute

12:10–1:25 p.m.   Lunch break

12:25–1:25 p.m.   Powerpoint/audio presentation Dan Burden, Executive Director, Walkable Communities, Inc.

1:25–3:05 p.m.   **Panel 3: Addressing Critical Issues in Increasing Physical Activity Through Travel and Land Use Choices** Paper moderators (Mindy Fullilove and Donald D. T. Chen, respectively)

1:25–2:15 p.m.   **Role of Safety and Security in the Built Environment** Paper author—Anastasia Loukaitou-Sideris, School of Public Policy and Social Research, University of California at Los Angeles

Commentator—Susan Saegert, Center for Human Environments, City University of New York

2:15–3:05 p.m.   **Social Equity and Environmental Justice** Paper author—Benjamin Bowser, Department of Sociology and Social Services, California State University at Hayward[1]

Commentator—Gary Orfield, Graduate School of Education, Harvard University

---

[1] This paper did not successfully complete the peer review process and was not published.

3:05–3:20 p.m.	Break

3:20–5:00 p.m.	**Panel 4: Role of Institutions in Increasing Physical Activity Through Transportation and Land Use Policies, Regulation, Education, and Training** Paper moderators (Robert B. Cervero and Steven N. Blair, respectively)

3:20–4:10 p.m.	**Institutional and Regulatory Factors Related to Non-Motorized Travel and Walkable Communities** Paper authors—Michael D. Meyer and Eric W. Dumbaugh, School of Civil and Environmental Engineering, Georgia Institute of Technology Commentator—Hank Dittmar, Reconnecting America, Las Vegas, New Mexico

4:10–5:00 p.m.	**Encouraging Cross-Disciplinary Curriculum and Training Programs** Paper authors—Elliott D. Sclar, Graduate School of Architecture, Planning, and Preservation, Columbia University; Mary E. Northridge and Emily M. Karpel, Mailman School of Public Health, Columbia University Commentator—Russell R. Pate, Department of Exercise Science, University of South Carolina

5:00–5:30 p.m.	**Rapporteur's Report and General Discussion** Cora Craig, Canadian Fitness and Lifestyle Research Institute, Ottawa; and Elizabeth Deakin, Department of City

and Regional Planning,
University of California, Berkeley

5:30 p.m.   **Adjournment**

WORKSHOP PARTICIPANTS

Rudayna Abdo
American Planning
   Association

Geoffrey S. Anderson
U.S. Environmental
   Protection Agency

Linda Bailey
Surface Transportation
   Policy Project

John Balbus
Environmental Defense

Debra Bassert
National Association
   of Home Builders

David Belluck
Federal Highway
   Administration

Hillary L. Burdette
Children's Hospital
   of Philadelphia

David Burwell
Prague Institute for Global
   Urban Development

Kelly J. Clifton
University of Maryland
College Park

Wendell Cox
Wendell Cox Consultancy

Andrew Dannenberg
Centers for Disease Control
   and Prevention

Allen Dearry
National Institutes of Health

Robert T. Dunphy
Urban Land Institute

John Fegan
Federal Highway
   Administration

Lisa Fontana-Tierney
Institute of Transportation
   Engineers

Steven P. Hooker
University of South Carolina

Richard Killingsworth
School of Public Health
University of North Carolina

Kathleen Rae King
Volunteers of America

Gerrit Knaap
National Center for
    Smart Growth
University of Maryland
College Park

M. Katherine Kraft
The Robert Wood Johnson
    Foundation

Kevin Krizek
University of Minnesota

Keith Laughlin
Rails-to-Trails Conservancy

Linda Lawson
Office of the Secretary
U.S. Department of
    Transportation

Nolan Lienhart
Office of Representative
    Earl Blumenauer
U.S. House of Representatives

Leslie S. Linton
Active Living Research
San Diego State University

Hani S. Mahmassani
University of Maryland
College Park

Barbara McCann
McCann Consulting

Rebecca S. Miles
Florida State University

Mary Elizabeth O'Neil
Yale University School
    of Medicine

Barbara J. Moore
Shape Up America

C. Kenneth Orski
Urban Innovations

Michael Pratt
Centers for Disease Control
    and Prevention

Daniel A. Rodriguez
University of North Carolina
Chapel Hill

J. C. Sandberg
Committee on Environment
    and Public Works
U.S. Senate

Jason Scully
Urban Land Institute

Karen Silberman
National Coalition for
    Promoting Physical Activity

Jessica Solomon
National Association
    of County and City
    Health Officials

Audrey Straight
American Association
    of Retired Persons

Phil Troped
Harvard School
    of Public Health

Dianne Ward
Department of Nutrition
University of North Carolina
School of Public Health

Sherry B. Ways
Office of Planning
Federal Highway
    Administration

Tracey Westfield
National Governors
    Association

Robert Whitaker
Mathematica Policy
    Research, Inc.

Clyde Woodle
Subcommittee on Highways,
    Transit and Pipelines
Committee on Transporta-
    tion and Infrastructure
U.S. House of Representatives

Deborah Rohm Young
Department of Kinesiology
University of Maryland
College Park

Lisa Zahurones
Institute of Transportation
    Engineers

Study Committee Biographical Information

Susan Hanson, *Chair,* is Landry University Professor and Director of the Graduate School of Geography at Clark University. She is an urban geographer with interests in gender and economy, transportation, and sustainability. She has published numerous papers and journal articles on the travel patterns of individuals and households in urban areas and on gender issues in local labor markets. Dr. Hanson has been an editor of three geography journals— *Economic Geography,* the *Annals of the Association of American Geographers,* and *The Professional Geographer*—and currently serves on the editorial boards of several other journals. She is a member of the National Academy of Sciences (Section 64) and is a Fellow of the American Association for the Advancement of Science, the American Academy of Arts and Sciences, and the Center for Advanced Studies in the Behavioral Sciences. She is a Past President of the Association of American Geographers.

Bobbie A. Berkowitz, *Vice Chair,* is Professor and Chair of the Department of Psychosocial and Community Health at the University of Washington's School of Nursing and an Adjunct Professor in the Department of Health Services at the University of Washington's School of Public Health. Dr. Berkowitz also serves as Director of the Robert Wood Johnson Foundation's Turning Point National Program Office, whose mission is to transform and strengthen the public health system in the United States by creating a network of public health partners across the country to broaden community participation in defining, assessing, prioritizing, and addressing important health issues. Her research interests include public health policy, determinants of health and population health outcomes, information technology, and the interaction and intersection of public health with other sectors, including community groups, the private sector, health care, and policy. Dr. Berkowitz is a member of the Institute of Medicine (IOM), Section 10, Other Health Professionals. She previously served as Cochair of the IOM Committee on Using Performance Monitoring to Improve Community Health. She is a Fellow of the American Academy of Nursing.

Barbara E. Ainsworth is a Professor in the Department of Exercise and Nutritional Sciences at San Diego State University. Her principal area of research is physical activity, including epidemiology, surveillance, and assessment, and environmental determinants of physical activity. Dr. Ainsworth also focuses on the physical activity needs and interventions directed at women and minorities. She is a fellow in the American College of Sports Medicine and an editorial board member of the *Journal of Physical Activity and Health* and the *International Journal of Nutrition and Physical Activity.*

Steven N. Blair is President and CEO of the Cooper Institute in Dallas, Texas. His research focuses on associations between lifestyle and health with emphasis on exercise, physical fitness, body composition, and chronic disease. Dr. Blair served as the first president of the National Coalition for Promoting Physical Activity and held the position of Senior Scientific Editor for the Surgeon General's Report on Physical Activity and Health. Dr. Blair also served as a committee member on the IOM study to Develop Criteria for Evaluating the Outcomes of Approaches to Prevent and Treat Obesity.

Robert B. Cervero is Professor in the Department of City and Regional Planning at the University of California, Berkeley. Before joining the faculty in 1980, he was a transportation planner in Los Angeles; Billings, Montana; Atlanta; and Norfolk, Virginia. Dr. Cervero has written extensively on such issues as transit and urban form, jobs–housing balance, joint development planning, and commuting. He is the author of several well-known transportation books, including *The Transit Metropolis, Transit Villages* *in the 21st Century, America's Suburban Centers, Paratransit in America,* and *Suburban Gridlock.* He was the principal investigator and primary author of the recent Transit Cooperative Research Program study on *Transit Oriented Development (TOD) in America.* Dr. Cervero serves on the editorial board of the *Journal of Public Transportation.* He is a Fellow of the Urban Land Institute and World Bank Institute and chairs the National Advisory Board of the Active Living Policy and Environmental Studies Program of the Robert Wood Johnson Foundation. Dr. Cervero was a member of the National Research Council (NRC) Panel on Transportation Options for Megacities in Developing Nations and the Committee on National Urban Policy.

Donald D. T. Chen is Founding Executive Director and CEO of Smart Growth America (SGA), a nationwide coalition of more than 100 partner organizations working to realize a shared vision of growth that protects the environment while developing the economy, advances social equity, promotes affordable housing and community development, and preserves farmland. Before helping create SGA, Mr. Chen was Research Director for the Surface Transportation Policy Project, Senior Research Associate at the Rocky Mountain Institute, and Researcher at the World Resources Institute. He cochairs the Board of the Environmental Leadership Program, is President of the Board of the Institute for Location Efficiency, serves on the Board of West Harlem Environmental Action, serves on the Advisory Board of *Grist Magazine,* is Vice Chair of the Congress for the New Urbanism's Transportation Task Force, and is an Associate Member of the Northeast Environmental Justice Network.

Randall Crane is Professor of Urban Planning in the School of Public Affairs and the Institute of the Environment at the University of California at Los Angeles. His research interests include urban environmental and development problems both in the United States and abroad, with a focus on behavior–built environment interactions. Among his current projects, Dr. Crane is studying sprawl and smart growth. He is coauthor with Marlon Boarnet of *Travel by Design: The Influence of Urban Form on Travel* (Oxford, 2001). Dr. Crane served on NRC's Committee on the Use of the Mexico City Aquifer as a Water Supply Resource.

Mindy Thompson Fullilove is Professor of Clinical Psychiatry and Public Health at the Mailman School of Public Health, Columbia University. Her research interests include community health issues such as AIDS, violence, and substance abuse in low-income communities. Dr. Fullilove is an expert in the field of qualitative research and community health and has published a number of articles and books, including *The House of Joshua: Meditations on Family and Place.* She also served on the Task Force for the Guide to Community Preventive Services, which examines issues from obesity and physical activity to cancer screening and diabetes management. Dr. Fullilove has been a member of the NRC/IOM Board on Children, Youth, and Families and has served on several other NRC and IOM committees.

Genevieve Giuliano is Professor in the School of Policy, Planning, and Development at the University of Southern California (USC) and Director of the USC/California State University Long Beach Metrans Transportation Center. Dr. Giuliano's research interests include the relationship between land use and transportation, transportation policy evaluation, travel behavior, and the role of information technology in transportation. She has published more than 100 papers and reports and has presented her research at numerous conferences in the United States and abroad. She is currently a member of two international research consortia and serves on the editorial boards of several professional journals. She is a member and former Chair of the Transportation Research Board (TRB) Executive Committee and is a National Associate of the National Academies.

T. Keith Lawton recently retired as Director of Technical Services in the Planning Department at Metro, the metropolitan planning organization for the Portland, Oregon, area. Mr. Lawton led the model development work at Metro, where he concentrated on bringing pedestrian environment variables into the modeling process. Most recently, he was involved in the development of activity-based models that consider daily activity schedules and use tours, rather than trips, as the unit of travel. Mr. Lawton was also involved in the federally supported activity-based model development known as TRANSIMS at the Los Alamos National Laboratories. He was on the Editorial Board of the journal *Transportation*. He is past Chair and a current member of TRB's Transportation Demand Forecasting Committee and past member of the TRB Committee to Review the Bureau of Transportation Statistics' Survey Programs and of the TRB Committee for the Evaluation of the Congestion Mitigation and Air Quality Improvement Program.

Patricia L. Mokhtarian is Professor of Civil and Environmental Engineering and Associate Director of the Institute of Transportation Studies at the University of California, Davis. Before coming to Davis, she spent 9 years in regional planning and consulting in Southern California. Dr. Mokhtarian specializes in the study of travel behavior. Her research has focused on the travel-related impacts of telecommunications technologies, attitudes toward travel itself, and the role of lifestyle and attitudes in the relationship between residential location and travel behavior. She is on the editorial advisory boards of *Transportation Research* and *Transportation* and is a past board member of the International Association for Travel Behavior Research. Dr. Mokhtarian serves on the Executive Committee of the University of California Transportation Center. She is a former member of TRB's Group 1 Council, former founding chair and member of the TRB Telecommunications and Travel Behavior Committee, and a member of the TRB Traveler Behavior and Values Committee.

Kenneth E. Powell is Chief, Chronic Disease, Injury, and Environmental Epidemiology Section, Division of Public Health, Georgia Department of Human Resources. The relationship between physical activity and health has been an important theme during his career as an epidemiologist. He initiated the Centers for Disease Control and Prevention's epidemiologic work in the area by consolidating the scientific literature and setting the public health research agenda. He is a Fellow of the American College of Physicians,

American College of Epidemiology, and American College of Sports Medicine.

Jane C. Stutts is Associate Director for Social and Behavioral Research at the University of North Carolina Highway Safety Research Center. Her areas of research include bicycle and pedestrian safety, older driver safety and mobility, drowsy and distracted driving, crash data analysis, and injury prevention. She has published numerous journal articles and reports in each of these areas. Dr. Stutts is a member of the editorial advisory board of *Accident Analysis and Prevention* and of the Association for the Advancement of Automotive Medicine. She currently serves on the TRB System Users Group Council and on the Safety and Mobility of Older Persons Committee. She is past Chair of the TRB Bicycle Transportation Committee and was a member of the Committee for the Conference on Transportation in an Aging Society: A Decade of Experience.

Richard P. Voith is Senior Vice President and Principal of Econsult Corporation, which provides economic consulting services to assist business and public policy decision makers. He is also the Executive Director of the Greater Philadelphia Transportation Initiative, an organization dedicated to transportation policy analysis and research in Greater Philadelphia. Before joining Econsult, Dr. Voith served as Economic Advisor, Senior Economist and Research Advisor, Senior Economist, and Economist at the Federal Reserve Bank of Philadelphia. He held the position of Adjunct Professor in the Real Estate Department of the Wharton School at the University of Pennsylvania. He was on the Board of Directors of the Southeastern Pennsylvania Transportation Authority and served as its Vice Chairman. Dr. Voith is an economist and expert in transportation and real estate economics, including the impacts of transportation and other policies on the real estate market and development patterns. He is currently a member of the editorial board of *Real Estate Economics,* the Research Committee of the Metropolitan Philadelphia Policy Center, and the Research Advisory Group of the Greater Philadelphia Regional Review. Dr. Voith is a member of the American Real Estate and Urban Economics Association.